# Hypnotically Enhanced Treatment for Addictions

*Alcohol Abuse, Drug Abuse, Gambling, Weight Control, and Smoking Cessation*

Joseph Tramontana, Ph.D.

**Crown House Publishing Limited**
www.crownhouse.co.uk
www.crownhousepublishing.com

First published by

Crown House Publishing Ltd
Crown Buildings, Bancyfelin, Carmarthen, Wales, SA33 5ND, UK
**www.crownhouse.co.uk**

and

Crown House Publishing Company LLC
6 Trowbridge Drive, Suite 5, Bethel, CT 06801-2858, USA
**www.crownhousepublishing.com**

**British Library Cataloguing-in-Publication Data**
A catalogue entry for this book is available
from the British Library.

**13 Digit ISBN 978-098235736-1**

**LCCN 2009927264**

Printed and bound in the USA

*Dedicated to My Loving Wife, Lynn,*
*and my Children, Jim and Jody,*
*of whom I am so proud.*

# Acknowledgments

To my clinical assistant, Traci Olivier, without whose meticulous editing and assistance with the technical aspects of constructing the manuscript, I would have been figuratively "up the creek without a paddle."

I also wish to take this opportunity to thank the American Society for Clinical Hypnosis (ASCH) for the excellent training opportunities which allowed me, first of all, to gain the confidence to incorporate hypnosis into my clinical practice. Thanks to all of the ASCH presenters and faculty over the years who have expanded and fine-tuned my clinical hypnosis horizons. Finally, thanks to ASCH for allowing me to become a faculty member and present the materials in this manuscript at the 2009 ASCH Conference and Workshops.

# Contents

# Introduction

In a recent article entitled "The Science of Addiction," Lemonick and Park (2007) noted that 18.7 million Americans, or 7.7% of the population, are dependent on or abuse alcohol. They reported an estimate of 2 million members in Alcoholics Anonymous. They estimated that 3.6 million people are dependent on drugs, and approximately 700,000 are undergoing treatment for addiction. They estimated 71.5 million users of tobacco products, including about 23.4% of men and 18.5% of women who smoke cigarettes. The article stated that 2 million American adults (0.67% of the population) are reportedly thought to be pathological gamblers, and that 4 million adults are addicted to food, with about 15% of mildly obese people being compulsive eaters.

I have been treating smokers and weight loss clients with hypnotherapeutic interventions since shortly after my first ASCH workshop in 1978, and at some point thereafter began using hypnosis as an adjunctive technique with alcohol, drug abuse, and compulsive gambling. Over the years, I have been acutely aware of the lack of literature regarding hypnotherapy with the latter three addictions. My focus is on patients who call or show up at an outpatient office requesting treatment for previously untreated or ineffectually treated alcohol, drug, or gambling addiction, in addition to smokers or those interested in weight loss.

What is the reason behind the dearth of literature and training opportunities on treatment of alcohol, drug and gambling addictions via hypnotherapy? There are likely several. Perhaps it is because hypnotherapists are reluctant to "step on the feet" of programs/philosophies such as Alcoholics Anonymous, Narcotics Anonymous, or Gamblers Anonymous. Perhaps it was because Milton Erickson (Erickson, 1976), who is so highly revered in the hypnosis field, stated that hypnosis was not a good approach for alcoholics because hypnosis encouraged: (1) an unhealthy negative transference, and (2) dependence on the therapist. One might find this quote strange in light of the fact that Haley (1985) reported conversations with Erickson in 1957 regarding several cases in which he successfully treated alcoholics. Of course, he was using what he referred to as a "strategic therapy" approach rather than formal hypnotherapy. In Rossi's (1980) four volumes on *The Collected Papers of Milton H. Erickson on Hypnosis*, there are absolutely no references in any of the four subject indexes on alcohol abuse, drug abuse, or gambling.

All of this is to say that the purpose of this book is, therefore, to offer new strategies, techniques, and scripts for use with problem drinkers, alcoholism, drug addiction, and gambling addiction in an outpatient population, as well as to review old and to present new techniques or combinations of techniques, strategies, and scripts for other addictions. The five addictions to be addressed are: alcohol abuse and dependency, drug abuse/addiction, gambling compulsions/obsessions and addictions, tobacco addiction (including cigars, pipes and chew), food addiction/compulsions. In the latter two, the "strategies and techniques" section will also address marketing and/or providing a package of sessions, with various preplanned scripts used in each session.

The title includes the term "hypnotically enhanced" versus "hypnotherapy" because, as the reader will note, many of the techniques and strategies incorporate a variety of therapeutic modalities, including: cognitive-behavioral techniques (Meichenbaum, 1977; Zarren & Eimer, 2002), solution-focused brief therapy (de Shazer, 1988), reframing and other NLP techniques (Grinder & Bandler, 1976), systematic desensitization, covert sensitization, techniques from the literature on "healing the wounded child within" (see Whitfield, 1987), 12-Step programs, guided imagery and meditation, among others. Furthermore, the techniques are employed both in and out of trance.

In the chapters on alcohol, drugs, and gambling, the reader will note that in not all of the sessions will hypnotic states even be induced or elicited. In the chapters on smoking cessation and weight loss, the time- or session-limited structure of the program will incorporate hypnosis into each session.

Additional points of note have to do with "hypnotic states" versus "trance" and "elicitation" versus "induction." Although the author may at times utilize the terms "trance" or "induction" loosely, "hypnotic state" and "elicitation" are preferred, for similar reasons. From an anthropological perspective, DePiano (2004) stated that "trance" could imply both "possession trance" in which someone loses conscious awareness and an invading spirit "takes over" with it's own behavior, speech patterns; and body movements or "trance," a so-called altered state of consciousness including the loss of conscious awareness but without the presence of a spirit or other outside entity. He adds that since a hypnotic practitioner is not an intrusive spirit or a sorcerer (I like to add, "At least, most of us aren't"), it makes more sense to talk about "the hypnotic condition," "hypnotic situation," "hypnotic process," or "the hypnotic experience" than about "the hypnotic trance." I prefer "the hypnotic state." So while I may occasionally call it a "trance," the goal is for patients to feel comfortable with the idea that hypnosis does not involve my controlling them, but rather that I will be teaching them to control themselves. So after considerable discussion of what hypnosis is and what it's not, the term "hypnotic state" seems preferable.

Likewise, "induction" implies something from outside going in, while "elicitation" implies bringing out what was inside, as was so aptly described by Zeig (2005) in a recent presentation. Again, the terms might be used interchangeably (i.e., "induction" for "elicitation," "trance" for "state"), and this is explained to the patient/client (also used interchangeably).

While there are some excellent books of hypnotic scripts in the literature (Allen, 2004; Hammond, 1990; Havens & Walters, 1989) which can be adapted to use with alcohol abuse or problem drinking, drug abuse, and pathological gambling, none have specific scripts for this client population. In summary, all of the strategies, techniques, and scripts herein have to do with helping clients take more effective control of their lives. As will be discussed in the chapter on alcohol treatment, the first Step in 12-Step approaches fosters the idea that the addicted client is powerless over alcohol (for example). This concept is somewhat antithetical to the approach most psychotherapists attempt to engender in their clients; i.e., take effective control of your life. In fact, Glasser, who a number of years ago began the Reality Therapy treatment approach, wrote a book titled *Take Effective Control of Your Life* (Glasser, 1984). Ways in which a slight modification of these words to be more consistent with psychotherapy will be presented.

A special word of note is offered here. As members of ASCH will attest, there is such "in-breeding" of teachers, trainers, and their students who become trainers, that many use similar techniques/ methods. Many of the techniques described in the subsequent chapters reflect a 31-year evolvement of techniques or blending of approaches; therefore, there may be places where the exact lineage of a concept or tool is no longer discernible. For example, after attending Mutter and Crasilneck's (2007) presentations at the ASCH/SCEH joint meeting in Dallas, I realized that I utilize many of their techniques, albeit heard or read about many years earlier. Likewise, in hearing Torem's (2007) presentation on weight loss, I realized that many of my techniques were similar to those he espoused, suggesting that I have heard him present these techniques in past years or have read about his work, without being consciously aware of the experience. However, my goal is to, whenever possible, give credit to those teachers, trainers, or contributors who deserve it, thereby honoring their contributions and providing readers with additional resources in their quest for knowledge.

After the appendices, there is an annotated resource list for further study or utilization.

# Chapter One

# *The Lens*

Let me begin by describing the way in which I understand psycho-therapy in general and more specifically the role of hypnotherapy within it. My view has evolved over the course of 39 years doing psychotherapy, the last 31 of which have included hypnotherapy. This evolution was in collaboration with hundreds of patients I have seen over those years.

As indicated in the Introduction, like many of my colleagues, I started using hypnosis with smokers and weight loss clients at first. As I became more proficient in the utilization of hypnosis as a technique to effect positive changes, I began using it for many other applications. These included (not in any chronological order): chronic pain patients to reduce subjective pain; stress/anxiety reduction; overcoming phobias; performance enhance-ment, including sports, study habits, exam taking; public speak-ing; recovering lost memories; uncovering subconscious reasons for self-sabotage; dealing with self-esteem issues by uncovering unconscious origins for feelings of low self-worth; uncovering early origins of sexual fetishes; decreasing habits such as scratch-ing infected skin or hair pulling (trichotillomania); working with bed-wetters; patients with Dissociative Identity Disorders (it was called Multiple Personality Disorder when I started); and last, but not least, with the topic of this book, patients with addictions.

Over the years, I have had great success with all of the above, or I wouldn't be writing about it (although I do note some failures). A few years ago, I gave an American Psychological Association approved continuing education presentation (Tramontana, 2005) at the Gulfport, MS VA Hospital entitled "Hypnosis as an adjunc-tive technique in psychotherapy." In that training seminar, a number of case studies were briefly presented covering most if not all of the above applications.

Harry Feamster, who has been retired quite some time, taught me a technique using aversive stimuli with problem drinkers (Feamster & Brown, 1963). Harry told me once: "Joe, hypnotherapy is the most economically efficient psychotherapy tool we have. It is quick and effective." Over the years I have found Harry right on target; that is, I can often find out as much in one hour of hypnotherapeutic uncovering as I could in many, many hours of traditional talk-type therapy.

A word about uncovering may help the reader understand how I use this technique. As explained in some of the later chapters, I use what I describe to the client as an "affect-bridge." I tell them that if we can uncover some early origin of the presenting problems, then it "bridges the gap", so to speak. I then indoctrinate them to the technique of hypnoprojection whereby they are imagining watching a movie of themselves in the past, so that they do not have to re-live the experience, just in case the experience was traumatic. In fact, they can describe it almost as if they were narrating a documentary.

As described in Chapter 3, my understanding of using hypnosis to treat drug abuse or addiction happened somewhat by accident. A young woman came in because her treating physician said that he had done all that he could to alleviate her back pain, but that if she could find someone who could teach her self-hypnosis, this technique would help. I thought: *What an enlightened soul!* After our first hypnotic session, I asked my typical post-trance question: "How do you feel?" She responded: "Damn, that was better than drugs!" It turned out that she was not talking about pain medications; rather, she and her husband used to do a lot of illicit drugs, mostly downers, such as Quaaludes and marijuana. I thought, "Hmm!" Especially for the population of clients whose drug of choice is one to quiet, mellow, or calm them down, hypnosis/self-hypnosis would be a valuable tool. And it is natural!

As the word got around that I was rather proficient at hypnotherapy, a number of clients with various addictions sought my services. As I describe in Chapter 2 on Alcohol Abuse and Problem Drinking, at first I was reluctant to treat alcoholics or drug addicts unless they agreed to attend a verbally contracted number of 12-Step meetings per week. Over time, I realized that I was excluding some people I might have otherwise helped who had trouble with AA/NA specifically or the group process in general. As a result, I became more flexible about this requirement. I was also impressed by Flemons (2002), who described how AA teaches clients that they can never trust themselves, and how this seems rather antithetical to psychotherapists' attempts to teach people that they can take effective control of their lives. So as time passed and experience grew, I became more flexible in developing treatment plans that would best suit the individual.

A short time before completing this manuscript, I had the good fortune of attending a CEU presentation by Dabney Ewin. While Dabney was presenting his ideomotor signaling technique, with a focus on working with patients with psychosomatic illnesses (Ewin, 2008), I came to realize how it might also be adapted to my work with addictions. My interest level was piqued, and I bought his book on this subject (Ewin & Eimer, 2006). This workshop also stimulated me to take another look at David Cheek's work (Cheek & LeCron, 1968; Rossi & Cheek, 1988). One case in which this approach was used with good results with a pathological gambler is presented in Chapter 4. A case in which Ewin's approach was successfully incorporated into a weight loss program is presented in Chapter 6.

## *Enter the Client*

When clients first come into my office, whatever the reason, they fill out a problem checklist and we briefly discuss the symptoms they have checked. Following that, I give them an overview of how I see therapy, using a coaching metaphor that came out of a session with a client.

> A number of years ago, I had a young man come in for his first psychotherapy session. I noticed from his information sheet that he had not been in therapy before. He was kind of fidgety and shuffling his feet. I asked him if he felt a little uncomfortable being there. He said: "Yeah man, I don't know if I'm wasting your time and mine." To which I responded: "I know, guys are supposed to solve their own problems, right?" He agreed, and

I continued, "And big boys don't cry, right?" Again he nodded in agreement. Well, luckily for me, it happened to be that time of year when the Summer Olympics were going on. Coincidentally, the Summer Olympics are on the same four-year rotation as the presidential campaigns for the November elections, so the races were heating up. I asked: "Did you read the newspaper today?" After he acknowledged he had, I asked: "Did you read about all of the Olympic athletes?" He responded: "Oh yes. I love the Summer Olympics!" I continued: "Did you read about all of the presidential candidates? I'll bet everyone you read about who was any good at anything had someone working with them behind the scenes to make them better. The athletes all have coaches. The candidates have advisors, campaign managers, and speech writers. Actors have directors. Anybody who is good at anything has someone helping him or her to get better. Mike Tyson was heavyweight champion of the world, before he got so crazy and started biting people's ears off. But even Mike had this little old guy in his corner reminding him to keep up his left, how to move, etc. Mike knows he is supposed to keep up his left, but sometimes it helps to have someone objective looking in and giving guidance … And that is how I see therapy. It is like having a coach, but one who coaches or consults with you regarding life's issues or problems you want to change."

This metaphor worked so well with this man that I began using it with others. The idea of a "coach" is accepted especially well by adolescents, and it is not gender-specific.

Another topic stressed in the opening session is the importance of being open. I explain to the client:

The therapist has only as much power to help as you give to him or her. And the way you give this power is by being honest and open. Now I know it is sometimes hard to open up to a total stranger, but for me to help, I have to know what I am really dealing with … A number of years ago, when I was director of a mental health center, I had an employee who was going through a divorce and needed therapy. She was also a friend. So I referred her to one of the psychiatrists who worked for us in one of our satellite clinics. I never breached privacy by asking her how the treatment was going, but one day I asked, "Are you still seeing F?" She responded: "You know, it is interesting you should ask. We just had our final session last week." I asked: "Well, did it help?" She answered: "Oh, I don't know; not really." I expressed my surprise: "Really, I always heard he was such a good therapist!" Her reply told the story: "Well, you know, Joe, he never did really know me." I responded: "You mean you went to

4

see that man once a week for six months and you didn't let him get to know you?"

The first session is also often when I talk with clients who come in seeking treatment for addictions about the "acting-out cycle." The idea is that when one engages in a behavior that causes feelings of guilt, embarrassment, or shame, the logical, rational response would be to say: "Well, I'm not going to do that again. I don't like the way I felt after doing that!" Often, however, the very behavior that caused the negative feelings arouses the person to a level of excitement (or calm) that gets them over the negative feelings. The high that comes with drinking, or drugs, or gambling, for example, helps one forget the previous negative feelings, and so the behavior continues to be repeated in a cyclical fashion. I explain this phenomenon so early in treatment because of what is often referred to in psychiatric hospitals as a "flight to health." Whether in a psychiatric unit or a substance abuse rehabilitation unit, patients often report after just a few days that they have learned the error of their ways, have "seen the light," and are "reformed." If they subsequently are successful in extricating themselves from the treatment facility, relapse is often quite rapid. The client is warned that the same issues arise in outpatient psychological treatment; therefore, I want at least a verbal commitment regarding continuing to work with me until we mutually agree on termination. As will be seen in the chapters on smoking cessation and weight loss, for those issues I have the client commit and pay for a package of sessions in advance. While I do not do that type of contracting with alcohol, drugs, and gambling, the intent is to let clients know that hypnosis is not a quick or magical cure, and that they will need to "stay the course" (a phrase from 12-Step programs) if we are to be successful.

Many patients come to my office specifically seeking hypnosis for addictive behaviors because they have seen my ad in the Yellow Pages or have heard about my treatment from others. In other cases, I am the one who mentions hypnotherapy as a possibility. It is interesting that even those who ask for hypnotherapy are sometimes quite skeptical about the procedure and whether or not they will be responsive to hypnosis.

When a patient reports that they do not know if they can be hypnotized, my standard answer is, "Oh, anybody bright and creative can be hypnotized." Not surprisingly, the client typically says, "Oh, okay." I tell the patient, "Only once has a client called my bluff, stating, 'Oh well, I guess that leaves me out!' As it turned out, she was a very bright (and witty) woman, and she was an excellent hypnotic subject." This response typically brings a chuckle from the client, thus enhancing rapport.

Regardless of why the patient wants to be hypnotized – whether to quit smoking, lose weight, deal with addictions, for pain control, as an adjunctive technique to other psychotherapy, or something else – I always start off by providing an overview. Even if the patient has been hypnotized by another provider in the past, this overview presents my particular philosophy about hypnosis and how it works. Typically, the patient is told that when talking about what hypnosis is, I often find myself spending a lot of time talking about what it is not. Many people only have the image of stage hypnotists who try to convince their audience that they can use hypnosis to control the minds of individual members of the audience, even to do silly things like crawl around like a chicken and cluck. A little education is called for:

> In medical and psychological hypnosis, the idea is that I can't control your mind, nor would I want to. But I can teach you to use your own mind power to achieve your goals. The key is that it is your mind power, not mine, so I serve only as a teacher or guide. You can't be hypnotized against your will, so we say that all hypnosis is self-hypnosis in a way. You have to be a willing participant. You have to want to do it.

The explanation continues:

> Hypnosis is an altered state of consciousness. It is not an unconscious state. The name is a misnomer. It comes from the Greek word *hypnos*, which in Greek means sleep. But you will not be asleep … you will be very much awake. Your eyes will be closed only to block out distractions, just like the music lover might put on headphones and close his or her eyes to focus more intently on the sound and block out visual distractions. You will hear everything I say. You'll be able to talk back if I ask you questions. You will remember everything we talk about, unless there is some reason to block it out. When your mind and body are totally relaxed, you can

concentrate better on everything I say … on whatever it is we are dealing with … in this case, suggestions about drinking (for example).

Depending on the situation, the patient may or may not be given a test of hypnotic suggestibility; instead, they may be given a muscle testing demonstration during which I say: "This is not hypnosis. This is a demonstration of the power of your mind." My first experience of this technique (Poulos & Smith, 1998) was later demonstrated by a number of other mental and physical health providers. I adapted this approach for my work with clients. In fact, I now use this muscle testing with almost all clients, even though hypnosis may never be part of their treatment plan. The client is told:

I want you to hold out one arm (the one closer to me), and as I describe something to you, I want you to make it very rigid and resist to the best of your ability when I try to push your arm down … Now, I want you to think about the greatest accomplishment of your whole life … something you are totally proud of that you would like everyone to know about. You would be happy to see it published on the front page of the local newspaper. Nod when you have something in mind. *Clients nod and invariably show great power to resist their arm being pushed down. Then the client is told to relax the arm for a while, after which they are told:* Now I'm going to ask you to make your arm rigid again … and now I'm going to tell you something else to think about. I want you to think about the lowest, most lowdown thing you have ever done in your life; something you are totally embarrassed about that you would not want anyone to know about … nod when you have it in mind … now resist. *Invariably the client's arm is easily pushed down. I then tell a story about when I used this technique as a demonstration to the athletic coaches at the University of New Orleans.* I had worked with a varsity volleyball player who after just three sessions had her best game ever. She was written up in the local newspaper as having her career high in "digs." I did not even know what a dig is but soon found out that it is a defensive "save." When the coaches learned that I had taught her self-hypnosis, they asked if I would give a presentation to the athletic department. I used this technique, asking for a volunteer from the audience. The women's basketball coach volunteered. He was not only tall, but very muscular. I whispered the first instruction (something you are very proud of) in his ear. I was practically hanging from his arm and couldn't budge it. Then I whispered the negative suggestion, and it immediately and easily went down.

On other occasions, such as when a patient comes in for a free consultation for a weight loss program [putting together and marketing weight-loss programs are discussed in Chapter 6], they might be given a little test of hypnotic suggestibility.

The goal is to show the potential client that they are likely to be a good hypnotic subject. Whether this test is done is often determined by the client's report of whether or not they have been previously hypnotized. Their degree of skepticism is also a determining factor. If the client acknowledges experience with hypnosis, they are asked their response to hypnosis. Time constraints may also be a determining factor as to whether or not a test of hypnotizability is employed. The test I most often use is one that I learned at one of my first ASCH workshops. The person is told to sit back comfortably in the chair, relax as much as possible, and when I say to put out their arms, to put both arms out, directly in front, at about shoulder height. I demonstrate the position and then continue:

> I want you to imagine a scene ... a beach scene. I want you to imagine sitting on a beach, on a beautiful spring or summer day. Perhaps you are sitting on a beach towel or blanket, or maybe a recliner of some sort ... enjoying the beautiful weather ... you feel the warm sunshine on your skin ... and a nice breeze coming off the ocean ... enjoying the beautiful scenery ... and imagine there are some children playing near the water's edge ... they could be children you know or could be strangers ... playing with their little sand buckets and shovels ... now when I was a child these buckets were usually made out of some kind of metal material, tin or aluminum ... nowadays they are typically rubberized or plastic ... but the one thing they still have in common is they all have the little curved handle so that the child can carry the bucket ... imagine that one of the children comes over to you asks you to put out your arms, so go ahead and do so now, just as I showed you ... then imagine that the child places the handle of the bucket over one of your wrists, whichever you decide, and then starts filling the bucket with sand ... and as the child does so, the bucket gets heavier and heavier ... the natural pull of gravity will cause that arm to gradually descend toward the ground, the sand below .... And you'd like to hold it up, but it gets heavier and heavier. It's now about one third full and getting really heavy ... and then the child starts filling it with wet sand, and wet sand is even heavier than dry sand because it is denser.

By then the arm is usually descended, or at least the client will report it feeling strained from holding up the bucket.

All of the above are part of the client's orientation to hypnosis. At this point (the first meeting) formal hypnosis has not commenced. I would like to note here that by design, different induction techniques are used as well as different deepening techniques. The first hypnotic session is often not until the actual second meeting. Because of my feeling regarding the importance of orienting the client to what we are doing and why, the first hypnotic session (typically the second actual meeting with the client) is very much structured and includes very specific techniques. An exception to this format is smoking cessation and weight loss clients, for whom I often start hypnosis in the first formal session because of the time-limited (packaging) techniques that are discussed in Chapters 5 and 6.

As will be seen in Chapter 2 on alcohol abuse and problem drinking, I often start the first hypnotic session with a reverse arm levitation technique, deep breathing techniques, followed by a deepening technique involving visual imagery of an elevator ride (unless the client has an elevator phobia) to a safe comfortable room. By design, different induction techniques are used in subsequent sessions. Such techniques include eye fixation, an eye roll approach, and progressive relaxation (imagined, not via progressive relaxation exercises). Sometimes, after patients are very experienced in working with me with a variety of techniques, I might say: *Just close your eyes and go into a deeper trance than you are already in.* I have come to realize that for some clients just sitting in my recliner has become a conditioned stimulus for trance induction. Further, with clients experienced in my approach, after the first three or four sessions, I will use what I refer to as "flex induction." In such cases, the client is told:

> You have been practicing a variety of induction techniques here and at home. Some clients prefer some methods and others prefer others! Now, just put yourself into a hypnotic state using whatever technique you like best.

Different deepening techniques are also employed. If I use the imagery of an elevator ride the first time, I might use a staircase, escalator, or gently sloping hill in subsequent sessions, always counting the client down. Later, I might even use counting forward as they imagine an escalator ride up into the clouds, each number taking them to a *higher level of relaxation ... where you can be above the humdrum of daily living and see things from a better perspective.* Again, after the client becomes experienced in my deepening techniques, I will do the same as with the induction:

> You have also been practicing a number of different deepening techniques both here and at home, so you pick whichever one you like best and allow yourself to go deeper now. Nod your head when you have completed the deepening technique in your mind.

The sessions typically go from more structured, detailed approaches to shorter, less detailed and more flexible ones. I prefer the reverse arm levitation technique in the first hypnotic session because this approach is slower and more dramatic than some of the others. While I am telling the client what is likely being felt in the arm and in the eyes, they actually feel the physiologic response of the arm getting heavier and the eyes getting heavier.

After hypnosis is elicited with the reverse arm levitation technique, some time is spent with diaphragmatic breathing. Then the client is told:

> Now, to get you more deeply relaxed, we are going to use a technique called visual imagery. Some people refer to this as visualization. I sometimes call it getting a picture in your mind's eye ... almost as if you had a screen back behind the eyes and the mind could see it.

If the client had previously experienced the beach scene imagery, I might reference that: *Just like with the beach scene ... you demonstrated that you are good at visual imagery.*

Following such confirmation, the client is presented with the next step:

> I want you to imagine yourself on the tenth floor of a building. This could be a building you have been in before or it could be one you've seen in a movie or on TV. But imagine there are ten floors. You are on the top floor, and you want to take an elevator ride all the way down to the first floor,

the bottom floor. Each floor, as you go down, is going to represent to you a deeper level of hypnotic relaxation. I want you to use all of your senses. See yourself, feel yourself, sense yourself going deeper with each number as I count. Starting with the tenth floor, imagine you are standing in front of the elevator doors, the doors open and you step inside. You turn around and face the front, and you see a control panel with ten buttons, one for each floor, plus a couple of others for opening and closing the doors. Let me know by nodding your head gently when you get a picture in your mind's eye of that control panel *(if the patient has difficulty, they are told to think about the last elevator they were in)* ... Now, I want you to imagine pushing the button that says one, and nod when you have done so ... good ... you pushed the button that said one and you are ready to start your descent ... You may notice above the doors often there is a set of lights and numbers, some way of monitoring your trip ... . So you've pushed the button and are ready to start down ... going down, from the tenth floor down to nine ... deeper to eight ... at seven going deeper ... every muscle and fiber in your body relaxing further with each number as I count ... six, and deeper ... at five you're half way down and with the remaining numbers letting go of all remaining tensions and relaxing very deeply ... at four ... three and deeper ... two ... all the way down to one, relaxing deeply ... and as you get to the bottom floor, imagine the elevator doors opening and you step into a hallway or corridor ... and from there into a room ... a very warm, safe, peaceful, comfortable room ... This could be a room you have been in before. It might even be your favorite room. Or it could be one you've seen in a movie or maybe in a magazine. Let me tell you how I see the room, and then you can either adopt my model or create your own ... ... I see it as warm, safe, peaceful, tranquil ... perhaps thick carpet on the floor, and a couch or easy chair, the kind you just sink down into and feel almost like you're part of the furniture ... see yourself entering the room, however you see it in your mind's eye, and walking over to the couch, or chair, or bed, or pillows, whatever furnishings are there, and really settling in ... sinking in ... becoming so deeply relaxed that it's hard to tell where your body stops and the furnishings beneath you begin ... and if you allow yourself, you can become just that relaxed right here, in this chair (or couch) ... so deeply relaxed it's hard to tell where your body stops and the chair beneath you begins ... appreciate how relaxed you're becoming ... appreciate how relaxed you've become ... in a state of perfect relaxation, you feel unwilling to move a single muscle in your body ... feel how good it feels to know that you don't have to move a single muscle in your body.

Next, the patient is instructed:

I'm going to tell you some things about hypnosis. You don't have to concentrate on what I'm saying, because your subconscious will pick it up anyway ... I'm going to tell you about two effects ... first, the "practice effect" ... just like most other behaviors, the more you practice, the better you get. So let me suggest to you that anytime you want me to put you into the hypnotic state, you will go into hypnosis more quickly and more deeply *(I typically repeat this suggestion three times)* ... And the same will hold true with the self-hypnosis that I will be teaching you to practice at home ... With practice, you will get better and better at putting yourself into a hypnotic state more quickly and more deeply ... The key word here is "want." I said: "When you want me to put you into hypnosis" ... neither I nor anyone else can put you into hypnosis against your will, and neither will you ever spontaneously go into a hypnotic state ... for example, while operating machinery or driving a car ... you will do so only when you want to ... only when it is to your advantage to do so ... the second effect is what I call the "generalization effect."

[This effect is really an ego-strengthening approach, which is to some extent a synthesis of Gregg's (1973) Analeptic Circle and Hartland's (1966) ego-strengthening techniques].

What I mean by generalization effect is that regardless of why you are learning hypnosis ... whether it is to stop smoking, lose weight, deal with chronic pain, deal with addictions, decrease stress, remember things from the past, improve sports performance or study habits ... you see, there are many applications of hypnosis ... the one common denominator ... or common fringe benefit, as I call it, is that you learn to be more calm and more relaxed ... because that is what the hypnotic state is all about ... learning to be more calm and relaxed ... and when you learn to be more calm and more relaxed, your functioning becomes more efficient and more effective ... and as you function more efficiently and more effectively, your self-confidence improves, leading to more calm and relaxation, even more effectiveness and efficiency, and even more self-confidence.

Since clients with addictions often feel that they have failed in many attempts to recover from the addiction, the goal is to reinforce a positive or optimistic forecast of success.

The importance of efficiency is explained a bit:

Many people, perhaps most people, expend much too much emotional energy, much more than the particular situation calls for ... this is what I

12

call spinning your wheels emotionally … as you learn to be more calm and more relaxed, you will engage in less of that emotional wheel spinning, and thus your functioning will become more efficient and more effective … And as you learn to function more efficiently and more effectively, your self-confidence improves, leading to even more calm and relaxation, efficiency, effectiveness, self-confidence, and so on … in a cycle of progress that grows, deepens, strengthens, and reinforces itself … this cycle of progress is like the so-called snowball effect … the little ball of snow that rolls down a hill and gets larger and larger as it gathers more and more snow … the end result of this cycle of progress is that you will have a better self-image, a better self-concept … what we call higher feelings of self-esteem … in other words, you will like yourself better, and you will be convinced that you can accomplish not only those things that you think you need to accomplish from day to day, but just about anything, within reason, that you set your mind to accomplish … and you will be able to do so calmly and relaxed, effectively and efficiently … with confidence.

After the generalization effect, I focus on trance ratification. As noted by Hammond (1990, p. 19), trance ratification is vitally important in creating a sense of expectancy in the client. This experience or experiences provide the client with a convincer that ratifies for them that they have entered into an altered state of consciousness. He describes glove anesthesia (p. 20) as one such technique. While I use his glove anesthesia technique with pain patients to demonstrate to them their ability to lower subjective pain, with most other clients I use three ratification techniques. The trance ratification techniques that I use follow:

Earlier I told you that you did not have to concentrate, because your subconscious would pick up what I was saying … but now, I am going to ask you to do just the opposite, because I want you to concentrate very intently on what I am saying. I want you to use the power of your creative mind, your imagination … and the first thing I want you to use your creative mind to imagine is that your eyes are glued closed … almost as if you had gotten some Super Glue or Crazy Glue or some such substance on the lids or lashes and you cannot open them … now as you imagine the eyelids glued closed, let the muscles in your eyes try to open them, but your mind is telling you that you cannot open them because they are glued shut … notice the resistance *(It has been very rare that a client opened his or her eyes)* … mind over matter … mind over body … now stop trying to open them … imagine the glue has worn off, but you decide to keep them closed until I tell you to open them…

13

After I have asked the client if it would be alright if I touch the arm nearest me, I say:

> I want you to place one arm out in front of you like this *(I help them line up the arm directly in front of them at shoulder height)* and make it very rigid ... That's right make a fist and make the arm very rigid, like a bar of steel ... an unbendable bar of steel ... you might even get a picture in your mind's eye of a bar of steel there instead of an arm ... tight and taut and unbendable *(I stroke arm with a finger and touch fingers around wrist to demonstrate)* ... and now, as your mind tells you that is an unbendable bar of steel instead of an arm, let the muscles of the arm try to bend it ... and notice the resistance there ... very good ... now I want you to imagine that the arm is no longer like a bar of steel ... instead, it is like a dishcloth *(I put fingers around wrist lightly)* ... limp and loose like a dishcloth.

The arm typically flops down beside the client. In fact, their response is one of the factors I consider regarding the client's hypnotizability. If they just gently lower the arm, it may be that the client is going along with what they think I expect. If the arm really drops like a dishcloth, this response indicates to me that they are truly in or entering into a hypnotic state. Then, depending on the particular application, appropriate suggestions follow (described in the following chapters).

In the second hypnotic session, the client is told:

> Last time, we created tension in the arm and in the eyes ... this time, we are going to localize the tension just in the eyes ... so I want you to stare at _____.

In one office, I had a picture of a candle high up on the wall, and I had the client stare at the flame of the candle. In other settings, I might just tell the client to pick a spot on the wall or ceiling that necessitates that they look up at an angle.

> ... This time we are localizing the tension just in the eyes ... and very quickly you will feel the eyes getting heavier and heavier ... this is called eye fixation, which is just a fancy way of saying "staring" ... and this causes the eyes to get heavier and heavier ... and whenever you are ready to let go of that tension in your eyes, all you need do is close the eyes comfortably and gently and relax further all over.

Once again, the induction is followed by diaphragmatic breathing exercises, and then a different deepening technique. A typical breathing exercise is introduced:

> I want you to take a really deep breath ... hold it ... and as you exhale, feel the tensions escaping from your body ... again, really deep breath ... now relax ... and again, deep breath ... and relax. Breathing is a key to relaxation. One of the things we know about human behavior is that humans are most relaxed when they are in a really deep sleep ... and during that deep sleep stage, peoples' breathing changes. It becomes very slow and very heavy. So I want you to breathe as you would in a really deep sleep ... slow and heavy ... slow and deep ... and each time you breathe in you might think ... in with relaxation, out with tension ... relax in ... tension out ... you might even feel lighter ... as if floating ... relax in ... tension out.

If the elevator image was used in the first session, the imagery of descending a staircase would likely be used in the second session. The exception is when the client indicates a fear of elevators, then I typically use the staircase imagery in the first session and move up the other imagery in subsequent sessions.

The client is told:

> Last time, we used the image of the elevator ride; this time we are going to use a staircase ... perhaps a spiral staircase, or perhaps one of those majestic staircases like in the old mansions, so long as each number symbolizes or represents to you a deeper level of hypnotic relaxation. I want you to use your senses ... see yourself, feel yourself, sense yourself going deeper with each number as I count ... starting with the tenth step and going down ... *The patient is taken from the tenth step all the way down to the first step.*

The third induction technique, which I usually introduce after the reverse arm levitation and eye fixation techniques have been utilized, is the eye roll technique. Again, the goal is to teach the client a variety of techniques so they can pick and choose the technique that seems to work most effectively. The eye roll approach is one I often recommend for the client to use in self-hypnosis, as it can be done just about anywhere, even when in public, by covering their brow with their hand. The patient is told in both the eye fixation and eye roll techniques:

We find that we can get more relaxed by creating tension in the eyes and then letting go, than we can by saying, "I think I'll close my eyes and relax now." It has to do with the difference between tension and relaxation, just like in the old progressive relaxation techniques in which people were taught to tense various muscles and then relax them. It is the contrast between tension and relaxation, which are mutually exclusive behaviors that teaches you to get more deeply relaxed.

Subsequent sessions might entail deepening techniques such as an escalator ride or descending a gently sloping hill down to an ocean or to a valley. When working with a client over several sessions, as described on page 10, I have them count forward from one to ten in an imaginary trip up into the clouds. This flexible approach helps increase the client's repertoire of techniques that they can use during their self-hypnotic work. Some clients have reported preferring this approach to counting down.

The client is told to practice at home, and at the end of the first hypnotic session, I teach a three-step self-hypnosis approach:

Step 1: Today I had you stare at a spot on your hand ... localizing the tension in both your eyes and your arm ... by next time, I will have you staring at a spot on the wall, localizing the tension just in the eyes. So this is what I want you to do at home ... *The client is then given the instructions for "eye fixation" as described earlier (for second session).*

... Step 2 involves the deep breathing as we described today. Unless people have breathing problems, they tend to take breathing for granted ... but if you can spend two or three minutes getting into your own breathing, breathing slow and deep, it is like getting into yourself, blocking out distractions ... Step 3 involves counting down, from 10 to 1, as we did today ... whether it is an elevator ride, an escalator ride, or descending a staircase or gently sloping hill, each number taking you more deeply relaxed ... then, you can review those things we worked on today ... now, if you are doing this at bedtime, you might give yourself the post-hypnotic suggestion that you are going to fall into a deep and restful sleep, not to awaken, unless, of course, there is an emergency, until the appointed time ... if you're doing it during the day, when you have other responsibilities, tell yourself ... I will continue relaxing for ___ minutes, whether it be 5 minutes, 1 minute, or even 30 minutes, depending on your other responsibilities, after which time I will open my eyes feeling wide awake, relaxed, refreshed, calm, and confident.

The particular application of hypnosis determines how many times per day a client is instructed to practice. I learned from Poulos and Smith (1998) that athletes are so used to practicing a lot of repetitions that they can be instructed to use self-hypnotic techniques many times a day. The same might hold true with alcohol and drug abusers. It is not uncommon for patients who go into inpatient treatment facilities for alcohol and/or drugs to be told that they need to attend 90 meetings in 90 days. So repetition may be familiar to this population. I have found that the client's willingness to practice at home is often a good predictor of motivation and of the likelihood of success. If the client reports that they are having trouble getting into a hypnotic state, I will often make a recording for them to use at any time, using suggestions tailored to the client's particular needs and using their name. I explain:

> What I call canned tapes … the kind you might buy in a bookstore, where everyone gets the same recording for every condition can be helpful, but I prefer to personalize the recording for your special needs.

In this chapter, I have presented my general approaches to hypnosis, along with some examples of induction and deepening techniques. The following chapters zero in on working with specific issues that respond well to hypnosis even as they seem intractable with other approaches. Also covered are guidelines on ways to get the word out about your work and how to market and grow your business.

## Chapter Two

# *Focus on Problem Drinking, Alcohol Abuse and Addiction*

This chapter presents an overview of the extent of the problems with alcohol. In addition, I outline my hypnotherapeutic approaches, including those that involve the traditional Alcoholics Anonymous (AA) goal of abstinence, as well as approaches to "controlled" or "social" drinking.

To state that alcoholism and problem drinking are expensive propositions is, of course, an understatement. They are expensive propositions not only with regard to the amount of money spent on alcohol for heavy drinkers, but also with respect to the potential loss of livelihood, relationships, and even freedom associated with it. The great cost across multiple dimensions has long been known by the business community. The forerunners of our current Employee Assistance Programs (EAPs) were called Occupational Alcoholism Programs. I co-authored a chapter many years ago on the assessment of the efficacy of occupational alcohol programs in a book entitled *The Treatment of Alcoholism in Industry* (Williams & Tramontana, 1977). Occupational Alcoholism Programs were developed by private industry to prevent or control the costs associated with loss of production, terminations, training new employees, and so on. The programs were later renamed in order to destigmatize them and to cover other problems under the same umbrella.

Alcoholics and problem drinkers seem to be especially attracted to hypnosis as a possible solution to their situations; perhaps they see it as their solution or "salvation." In general, addicts seem to be looking for the "quick fix" and for someone outside of themselves to "fix them." Early on in my work with alcoholics (and drug addicts), I would tell them that I could use hypnosis to help them relax and help them focus on "working their steps";

however, I would only work with them if they agreed to attend X number of AA meetings per week. In more recent years, however, especially with the increase in popularity of approaches such as Moderation Management (MM), I also work with patients who want to attempt to control their drinking rather than abstain entirely.

The MM approach asks the patient to agree to not drink more than four days/nights a week and to not consume more than three (for women) or four (for men) drinks on any of those four days/nights. The gender difference is based on average weight differences between men and women. It is also recommended that people who embark on this program abstain completely for a period of time to "clean out their system" before attempting to learn to control their drinking. Those who are dependent on alcohol or require detoxification would not be good candidates for this approach anyway. Other people who would not be candidates for this approach are those who, when they drink alcohol, are typically led to one of the other problems described in this book, such as drug abuse, pathological gambling, or addictive problems not addressed in this book, such as sexual perversions or addictions.

Moderation approaches are controversial to addictions counselors, for whom training and experience is based almost entirely on the 12-Step, 30-day (or longer) rehabilitation approach, but there is some recent evidence to support reconciling these approaches in some cases. As Flemons (2002) so aptly noted in his book *Of One Mind*, "Some therapy models, such as Alcoholics Anonymous, rely on teaching clients how they can never trust themselves. Whenever possible, I head in the opposite direction, encouraging people to trust their guts, their hope, fingers, voices, reservations and negative experiences." However, his last phrase, "negative experiences," is very important. One should not forget people's past failures in attempting to "control" their drinking rather than abstain.

Managed care, as much as it is despised by many healthcare providers, led to Individualized Treatment Plan approaches with alcohol and drug addicts. The episodic excessive drinkers, who occasionally or even regularly get drunk at parties or on holidays;

weekend alcoholics; or daily excessive drinkers appear to be quite different than those who drink chronically. Yet in the past, everyone received the same treatment. Although the dynamics of addictions may have some similarities, "not all drunks are created equal." The Sobells' book (1993) suggested that many problem drinkers could learn to be social drinkers, especially certain males who, as they became more mature, no longer hung around in bars with their buddies. Moderation Management has become an increasingly popular approach in recent years. The book by Rotgers, Kern, and Hoetzel (2002) entitled *Responsible Drinking* describes in great detail the moderation management approach.

My philosophical belief is that treatment should be goal-directed, but that the goals should be patient-directed. First of all, as noted above, hypnosis or hypnotherapy is a very attractive approach for addicts. For example, a client might call and/or show up for the first session asking, "Can you hypnotize me to help me quit drinking?" In such cases, the client is informed that hypnosis is not a "magical cure," although Shapiro (2005) suggested that sometimes the idea of "magic" is not a bad thing in terms of "expectancy." The client is then told: *However, I would be happy to work with you and teach you techniques to help you become sober and maintain sobriety.*

As is consistent with much of the ASCH training, we are taught to be permissive in our treatment (e.g., "Would it be okay if we do ____?"). Citrenbaum, King, and Cohen (1985) note that some addicts "require a kick in the ass" in order to get them to actively participate in the treatment. However, even with this population, I prefer to give the client a choice between complete abstinence or a moderation management approach, when possible. The exceptions to the rule are rare and dramatic; for example, the patient who presented with a distinct yellow tone secondary to the beginning of liver disease. Other exceptions would include individuals whose drinking repeatedly puts them into dangerous situations such as driving under the influence (DUI) or people who become violent when drinking, or are on court-ordered probation and randomly tested for alcohol intake. These and other conditions would make MM a poor choice. When given a choice, the problem drinker is likely to choose moderation over abstinence, and so in the absence of mitigating circumstances, the treatment goal will be to assist the client in achieving controlled drinking. If such attempts fail, however, an abstinence goal may become the only option. Further, I never attempt to influence a client to choose the moderation approach if they are already leaning in the direction of abstinence. Even AA proponents say, "If you think you can drink socially, experiment. If you are successful, good for you." The implicit message, of course, is: "You'll be back!"

I do not typically "test" the patients/clients formally when they come in for treatment for alcohol abuse or problem drinking. If doing a formal evaluation for other purposes, I might administer the Michigan Alcohol Screening Test (MAST) or Substance Abuse Subtle Screening Inventory (SASSI). If a client expresses a desire to know how they might score on standardized tests, for example, to see how they compare with normal versus problem drinkers, these assessment techniques will be used. Sometimes this information might be relevant in determining whether abstinence or moderation as a treatment goal is indicated. More recently, I have suggested to clients that they go to an alcohol screening website (www.alcoholscreening.org) to get feedback regarding the degree of harmfulness of their drinking routine. The site also offers a comparison of the percentage of the general population and the percentage of individuals in each gender who drink fewer drinks.

# 1. Abstinence Model

When abstinence is identified as the goal, I let the patient know that I will work with them to attain abstinence, but that I would prefer that we do so in conjunction with AA meetings. We then negotiate how many meetings per week. As noted earlier, in past years, I often would refuse to see patients who did not agree to go to AA. However, it soon became apparent that there were some patients who were so against group work, or who had tried AA in the past and felt very uncomfortable with it, that to be unyielding in that requirement might reject people who could, perhaps, be helped, even without the meetings. Following a determination of whether or not the client will incorporate AA into their treatment program with me, an overview of hypnosis is given, followed by muscle testing (as described in chapter 1, p. 7), and often a test of visual imagery (Chapter 1, pp. 8–9). The following techniques are used with clients for whom abstinence is the goal.

## The First Hypnotic Session

Since the first meeting with the client is usually for information gathering and developing a treatment plan, the second actual physical meeting is typically the first hypnotic session. A reverse arm levitation induction is used, followed by deep breathing exercises, and a deepening technique. Usually, the elevator metaphor is used in the first session. The induction is as follows:

> I want you sit back comfortably. Let's get your feet up. I want you to settle back and relax to the best of your ability. And as you relax in that manner, I want you to place one arm out in front of you, at about shoulder height *(I demonstrate)* like this … and keep that arm kind of loose and limp so that it is not locked into place *(if it continues to look rigid, I will ask:* "Is it alright to touch your arm?"*) Then I will demonstrate as I say,* "Let's bend it a little so it is not locked into place." … Okay, now I want you to stare at a spot on that hand, either one of your knuckles or fingernails, or your ring *(if they are wearing one)*. Focus on that spot and nothing else. And as you stare at that spot, your arm is going to feel heavier and heavier. The natural physical, physiological response is for that arm to feel heavier … the natural pull of gravity will cause it to feel heavier and heavier … your eyes will feel heavier and heavier … the natural response to staring in that manner is for the eyes to feel heavier and heavier … and you will wish to close them. You might feel a slight burning sensation or tearing sensation, and the need to blink more frequently … in fact, you have already started to blink more frequently, and with each blink, notice your eyelids getting heavier and heavier … and as soon as your arm touches down, whether it touches your leg, your lap, or the chair, that is your signal to yourself and to me that you are ready to let go of all tensions and relax further all over … and what we are doing now is localizing the tension in your arm and in your eyes … and what is really neat about this technique is that when you can localize the tension … place it where you want to place it, that puts you in control of that tension, in charge of it, meaning that you then also have the power to let it go whenever you are ready … *If the arm is already descended by then, I proceed to deep breathing exercises. If not, I say:* And you are probably curious about just how long

this will take ... and the answer is that you are in charge of that ... you are in control ... you can hold onto that tension for as long as you want or you can let it go as soon as you want ... you are in charge of that. *In the rare instances in which the arm is not descending, I say:* Even though your arm is bent, it seems rather locked into place ... so I want you to notice how each time as you inhale, the arm raises just a fraction, and as you exhale, it descends a fraction ... you might make a conscious effort to allow it to descend a little more each time you exhale than it went up the time before. *Typically this approach will finally result in the arm touching down. In even rarer situations in which the arm is still not down, I say:* Well, it still seems somewhat locked into place. So I'm going to help you with that ... *And I gently push down on the forearm until the arm touches down. I then get the client to focus on their breathing ... I say:* I want you to take in a really deep breath ... and hold it ... and now exhale slowly ... and again, deep breath ... hold it ... and now relax ... breathing is a key to relaxation ... one of the things that we know about human behavior is that humans are most relaxed when they are in a really deep sleep ... and in that deep sleep state, people breathe more slowly and more deeply ... so I want you to imitate that breathing pattern ... breathing like you would in a really deep sleep ... very slow and very deep ... that's right ... slow and heavy ... And each time as you take that really deep breath, you might think the word "relax" and as you exhale you think of any remaining tensions escaping from your body ... so it is in with relaxation, out with tension ... you might even tell yourself, "relax in, tension out ... relax in, tension out." *When the client seems to be breathing comfortably, I say:* Next I want you to focus on getting even more deeply relaxed ... we call this a "deepening technique."

I then introduce a deepening technique. As described in Chapter 1, pp. 10–11, in the first hypnotic session I typically use the visual imagery of an elevator ride from the tenth floor down to the first floor. Once the patient is in a relaxed state, the following hypnotic suggestions are given.

We have been concentrating on relaxing your body, and now let's relax the mind, as well. One way to relax the mind is to think of nothing for a while. Now it is not so easy to think of nothing. But one way to do it is to imagine that your mind is like a blackboard, or perhaps a computer screen, and you can just erase your thoughts and make it blank, letting your mind drift comfortably. You don't have to concentrate on what I am saying, because your subconscious mind will pick it up anyway.

Then we discuss the "practice effect" and then the "generalization effect," as indicated in Chapter 1, pp. 12–13. The practice effect relates to the patient the importance of practicing the self-hypnotic approaches that I will teach them for this program to have maximum effectiveness. The generalization effect is basically a method of boosting self-esteem and self-confidence. Confidence building is especially important with people who have addictions because usually they have tried to change many times, with limited or no success.

With alcoholics and problem drinkers, I always strive for deep levels of relaxation in the first hypnotic session, so they are given relaxing scenes to imagine, as follows:

> Now let's concentrate on getting even more deeply relaxed, and we are going to do this by having you imagine some relaxing scenes. The first scene I want you to imagine is a beach scene, or if not a beach, perhaps on the ocean so you could be on the sand or grass, and I want you to imagine yourself sitting on a beach towel, a blanket, or a recliner of some sort and really enjoying the weather, the scenery … Perhaps it is a beautiful spring or summer day … Feel the warm sunlight on your skin, with a nice breeze coming off the water. You are really enjoying the weather and the scenery, watching some sailboats off in the distance. It is a relatively calm day and you notice how effortlessly they seem to move through the water, pushed by the gentle breeze … Perhaps there are some seagulls flying nearby … near the water's edge, and you notice how they, too, seem to glide so effortlessly on the wind currents … and perhaps a ship on the horizon … Now we know that it takes a lot of power to motor a ship, but it is the efficient use of power that causes this seeming effortlessness … perhaps a jet plane in the sky. It too takes a tremendous amount of power, but once again, it is the efficient use of power that causes this seeming effortlessness. These are your key words, "efficiency and effortlessness."

> Now let's go to a second scene. This could be a scene in the woods, perhaps a state park-type setting. Perhaps it is a beautiful fall morning, one of those fall mornings where there is a nice sunlight, but you feel that certain crispness in the air … and you are walking down a path in the woods, really enjoying the scenery … the leaves are turning colors, birds are chirping, and you are enjoying the sights and sounds and smells of the forest … And as you are walking along the path, you notice an area ahead in which there are no trees … and as you get closer you see the

reason that there are no trees is that there is a body of water running through there, like a narrow river or wide stream, and you notice how effortlessly the water seems to flow, clean and clear, so crystal-clear you can see your image, your reflection, in the water. And you might see your reflection as you were at some younger age, some time before you developed the problems that led you to where you are now ... you notice how steadily the water flows ... how predictably, reliably efficiently and effortlessly . There are those words again ... efficiency and effortlessly ... Perhaps there are some rocks and pebbles near the water's edge, where the water is only an inch or two deep, and you notice how the water just kind of goes over or around these rocks or pebbles ... Perhaps there are some boulders protruding out in the stream and you notice how there, too, the water just goes over or around and continues on its path, effort-lessly. You continue to walk down the bank of the river or stream and you come upon a bridge ... a walking bridge ... the kind you might see in a state park ... a wooden bridge, with the curved hand rails, some people call them footbridges ... and you decide that you want to cross over to the other side. So you step up onto the bridge and start to walk across ... And as you get halfway across, you notice that something below has gone awry ... The water below is getting muddy and dirty and backing-up. It is not flowing so smoothly anymore. And as you look more closely, you see that apparently what has happened is some logs were floating down this body of water and they got lodged under the bridge, causing a log jam. As you investigate even more closely, you see that there is one log that is bigger than the rest ... It is the main problem. It got wedged under the bridge causing the others to back up behind it ... I want you to really concentrate on that big log. Some people, when they concentrate on that big log, might imagine something written on that log, written or engraved, or inscribed on that log. It might be a word or it might even be a name. It could be a sentence or even a full paragraph ... nod when you get some-thing ... *(if no nod, I say):* It is not essential that you see something, but regardless of whether you do or not, what is most important is the next step ... you make a commitment to take matters into your own hands to free up the problem ... to remedy the problem, and so you cross over to the other side and you find a board or a pipe or a tree limb, something you could use as a lever ... and you set about the task of freeing up the log jam. Whether it involves leaning over from the bridge, leaning out from the bank, or even wading into the water, you use that board, pipe or tree limb as a lever to pry loose that big log. And to your surprise, with a little effort, it begins to loosen up, and as it loosens, it starts to float again under the bridge ... and the other logs follow suit ... You go back up onto the bridge and you watch as the logs float off into the distance ... and the farther away they get the smaller they seem, and the smaller they seem the farther away they are until they are so very far away they are like little tiny specks in the distance ... And finally, they round a bend; you know they still exist somewhere, but they are no longer in your field of experience ... you look back down into the water and you take great pride in the fact that the water is once again flowing smoothly, cleanly, reliably, predictably. You see your reflection again, but this time you see yourself at your present age, in the here-and-now, as an adult, but you see yourself as looking much healthier, like the younger person that you saw in the beginning, free from the addiction ... And you take some pride in the fact that you took matters into your own hands to rectify, to remedy this problem ... Now, as you may have already figured out, this is a metaphor filled with symbolism ... The body of water symbolizes your path through life and that is why we showed you at an early age clean and clear and free. The little rocks and pebbles symbolize minor setbacks ... minor frustrations ... Of course the boulders represent bigger problems; the log jam, however, represents a major blockage, probably the addiction that led you to seek treatment ... some people see something written on the log that might give them a clue ... by the way, did you see something written on the log? ... *If yes, find out what the person saw. If not ...* and some don't, as I said. Some might see a name, some might see their own name, realizing that they are their own biggest problem, but the key is the decision to take matters into your own hands to free up the log jam ... which could be symbolic of coming to see me ... and perhaps I am, or hypnosis is, the lever ... the board ... the pipe or tree limb.

Next, we proceed directly to the 12 Steps. Initially, the 12-Step programs were developed by the forefathers of Alcoholics Anonymous and are now being used in virtually every effective self-help group that addresses addictive-compulsive or co-dependent behavior, from Narcotics Anonymous and Gamblers Anonymous to Overeaters Anonymous; from Al-Anon to Nar-Anon, Sex Addiction, and Co-Dependency. All of these groups incorporate the 12-Step program.

The patient is told:

"You are now ready, or you wouldn't be here in my office, to take Step One. You notice that the steps are written in the past tense, and that is because a group of people, who tried every other way, found, through experience, that these steps worked for them, so it is not an "I" program as much as a "we" program, and it is past tense.

STEP ONE: We admitted that we were powerless over alcohol, that our lives had become unmanageable. For all the other dependencies, you could fill in the appropriate word. For example, many people will need to admit that they were powerless over food, powerless over sex or lust ... For Co-Dependency, the first step is changed to "we admit" that we were powerless over our dependencies, that our lives have become unmanageable. Step One is the most difficult of all steps because so many people are in such denial of their addictions or co-dependencies. They tend to think, "We can handle it on our own." But usually they haven't done a good enough job. In some form or fashion, their lives are out of control; thus, their lives have become unmanageable ... So Step One ... we admitted that we were powerless over alcohol, that our lives had become unmanageable. *[I sometimes change this, depending on the patient's philosophical bent. For example, I would not change anything if his or her belief was totally entrenched in the 12-Step model. For others, I might tweak the wording. For example, "I came to admit that I am powerless when I drink," or "I came to admit that I am powerless over my drinking behavior," thus focusing on the out-of-control behavior rather than the substance.]*

STEP TWO: Once we have admitted our powerlessness, the next step is as follows: "We came to believe that a power greater than ourselves could restore us to sanity." And of course, this step remains constant regardless of the addiction. We came to believe that a power greater than ourselves could restore us to sanity. Now, of course, this step is where we get into a more spiritual aspect, although for some people who are not into spirituality, a power greater than themselves may be their 12-Step group, or their therapy ... a friend told me about a man who had always complained about the mention of God until one day he had a revelation. He suddenly realized that his higher power was GOD! G-O-D for group of drunks. So Step Two ... we came to believe that a power greater than ourselves could restore us to sanity ...

STEP THREE: We made a decision to turn our will and lives over to the care of God as we understand Him (or for those individuals who prefer, made a decision to turn our will and our lives over to the care of this higher power, as we understood him/her/it). Now, of course, it is hard to escape the spirituality of this step. The reason the early founders described it as such (i.e., "as we understand Him,") is because a lot of people who are atheistic in their beliefs would not have the benefit of AA or other addiction programs if this step would turn them off. Most people who are successful in the program find it to be a very spiritual one, at some level, at whatever level they are comfortable with ... so Step Three, again ... we made a decision to turn our will and our lives over to the care of God as we understand Him ...

The client is then brought out of the hypnotic state and taught a three-step self-hypnosis technique to practice at home. They are given suggestions about how many times a day to practice and regarding post-hypnotic suggestions to give themselves. The self-hypnosis training I teach is as follows:

> I want you to practice a three-step technique at home. Today, I had you stare at a spot on your hand, localizing the tension in the arm and in the eyes. In the next session, I will have you localize the tension just in the eyes, by staring at a spot on the wall or ceiling. So at home, I want to get into a comfortable position in a chair, couch, bed, wherever you are least likely to be distracted, and pick out a spot on the wall or ceiling that causes you to look up at an angle. This is Step 1! The more severe the angle, the more quickly will you feel the tension building in your eyes. This technique is called "eye fixation." Eye fixation is just a fancy term for staring. And when you feel that tension building in your eyes, that is your signal to just close the eyes and let go of the tension. And we find that when we create the tension in the eyes and then let it go, we can get more deeply relaxed than if we simply say: "I think I'll just close my eyes and relax." It has to do with focusing on the difference between tension and relaxation. Step 2 involves deep breathing ... just as I showed you today, breathing slow and heavy ... unless people have a breathing problem, they tend to take breathing for granted. But when you slow it down, breathing for 2 or 3 minutes just as you would in a deep sleep, it is a way of getting into you and blocking out external distractions. Step 3 involves using visual imagery and counting yourself down from 10 to 1 ... today we used the image of an elevator ride ... in future sessions we will likely use other images such as descending a staircase ... or an escalator ... or perhaps a gently sloping hill down to a beautiful valley or river ... as long as each number symbolizes to you a deeper level of hypnotic relaxation.

## *The Second Hypnotic Session*

After some discussion about the patient's experiences since the first session – including successes, pitfalls, and questions – a hypnotic state is again elicited. Typically, this takes the form of an eye fixation approach, followed by deep breathing exercises, and then a staircase metaphor (See Chapter 1, p. 15) for deepening. Next, the first three steps, as presented in Session 1, are reinforced. Next, the patient is told:

Last week, we focused only on Steps 1 through 3. Today, we will give you a hypnotic view of the other 9 steps (Steps 4 through 12), as well.

STEP FOUR: We made a searching and fearless moral inventory of ourselves. This is a very difficult step that many newcomers find challenging, because it involves a great deal of personal honesty, breaking down all denials and admitting to ourselves by working through this inventory all of our past wrongs. There are many good workbooks available to assist people in completing this difficult step.

STEP FIVE: Admitted to God (or a higher power), to ourselves, and to another human being the exact nature of our wrongs.

STEP SIX: We were entirely ready to have God (or our higher power) remove all the defects of character.

STEP SEVEN: Humbly asked Him to remove our shortcomings.

STEP EIGHT: Made a list of all the persons we have harmed and became willing to make amends to them all. It is important to know that Step Eight does not involve making amends ... It states that "we became willing to make amends."

STEP NINE: Made direct amends to such people, whenever possible, except when to do so would injure them or others. So Step Eight involves making a decision to make amends and Step Nine involves following through with it.

STEP TEN: This is somewhat of a continuation of Step Four; we continued to take personal inventory, and when we were wrong, promptly admitted it.

STEP ELEVEN: Sought through prayer and meditation to improve our conscious contact with God (or higher power) as we understand him/her/it, praying only for knowledge of His (or the higher power's) will for us and the power for us to carry it out.

STEP TWELVE: Having had a spiritual awakening as a result of these steps, we tried to carry this message to others and to practice these principles in our daily lives.

To summarize: ... People who are successful in these programs often find that they must do Steps 1, 2, and 3 every day. So, perhaps in a morning prayer or meditation, in conjunction with a self-hypnosis, we say that we admit that we are powerless over alcohol and that our lives have become unmanageable ... that we came to believe that a power greater than ourselves could restore us to sanity, and that we made a decision to turn our will and lives over to the care of God (or higher power) as we understood him/her/it.

## The client is told:

Step 4 seems to be more of a project than the others for most people. Steps 5, 6, 7, 8, and 9 are all connected. In Step 4, we are making the searching and fearless moral inventory and then in Step 5 we are admitting it to a higher power, to ourselves, and to another human. In Step 6, we decide that we are entirely ready to have God or a higher power remove all the defects of character, and in Step 7 we humbly ask him/her/it to remove our shortcomings. In Step 8, we made a list of anyone we had harmed, became willing to make amends and then in Step 9 carried through with his will by making such amends, except when doing so would injure them or others.

Steps 10, 11, and 12 are techniques developed to attempt to prevent relapse, which involves continuing to take personal inventory and when we are wrong promptly admitting it. In other words, once we have made the searching and fearless moral inventory in Step 4, and we have gone all the way through to making amends, it doesn't mean that we can start fresh with wrongdoings. We, therefore, continue to take this personal inventory. We seek through prayer and meditation to improve our conscious contact with a higher power, as we understand it, praying only for the knowledge of His (Her or its) will for us and the power to carry it out. And having had a spiritual awakening as a result of these steps, we try to carry this message to others and to practice these principles in all of our affairs. Many people in the program find that one of the primary things that keeps them sober, keeps them from relapsing, is what is called service work, which is to help others ... that is, to carry the message to others.

## The client is told:

All of these steps are now to be considered post-hypnotic suggestions to assist you in preparing to work these 12 Steps. For most people, it takes a considerable time to work through each step, and it helps to have a sponsor to work with you on them. In no way are these suggestions intended to take the place of or substitute for actual participation in 12-Step programs. The 12-Step programs are the most successful that we have for recovery and preventing relapse. Today's session and the hypnotic suggestions included are geared to help support and reinforce what you do in your own 12-Step program. Recovery is no easy task, but many tens of thousands have recovered through these programs ... and so can you. God bless you!

The client is then brought out of the hypnotic state awake ... relaxed ... refreshed ... calm ... and confident, especially ... very confident. The client is told: If you are practicing these techniques at bedtime, you will tell yourself,

"I am now going to fall into a deep and restful sleep, not to awaken ... unless, of course, there is an emergency ... until the appointed time (whether it is by alarm clock, sunlight in the room, etc.) and at that appointed time, my eyes will open and I will feel relaxed ... refreshed ... calm ... and confident, especially ... very confident.

So, Hypnotic Session Number 1 is a presentation of the first three steps of AA. Most important in the early stages are the first three steps. In Session Number 2, after discussion of their progress to date, successes, and problems, a hypnotic state is elicited. Then, a more intense approach to reinforcing the first three steps ensues, followed by an overview of all 12 steps.

In Session Number 3 and subsequent sessions, after discussion of their progress to date, as well as problems, other therapeutic techniques including those mentioned in Chapter I might be utilized. For example, the client's self-destructive tendencies might be approached through hypnotic regression. A variety of cognitive behavioral and insight-oriented approaches might be employed, hypnotically, to assist the client in obtaining a better understanding of his or her problem drinking.

One of the stories I tell clients, typically with the client in an alert state follows:

Step Nine, making amends, is often a difficult one. I heard an AA old timer speak about this once. He said that he had been presiding over a meeting in which a young man questioned: I know I have to make amends to my father, because I did some pretty rotten things to him. But he also did some even worse things to me. How do you make amends to someone you would really like to slap the shit out of?" The response was pretty simple: "Think about anyone you have ever felt that way about. They have probably already been hurt a lot worse than you could ever hurt them!"

# 2. *Moderation Management Model*

The Moderation Management (MM) model is gaining increasing popularity. As noted earlier, it is geared toward controlled drinking. In sessions with individuals opting for this strategy, a variety of psychotherapeutic approaches are employed. Further, some of the same approaches used with those who strive for abstinence are used, including cognitive-behavioral strategies to work with self-destructive strategies and hypnotic behavioral rehearsal techniques. A client, for example, will imagine being in various social settings that involve drinking and terminating their drinking once they have reached the limit.

There are two basic approaches to Moderation Management that I recommend to clients, both of which can be researched by the client on the internet. The first, "Moderation Management," can be found at www.moderation.org. The Moderation Management Approach involves either actual meeting sites or online support groups. As of the March, 2009 revision of the listings, there can be actual face-to-face group meetings in 14 states plus D.C. and Toronto. [See the Resource List and Recommendations for Further Reading.]

Another recommended moderation program is Alcohol Management. The website for this program is http://www.med. umich.edu/mfit/alcoholmanagement/index.htm. It is described as a brief, confidential educational program that helps one eliminate drinking problems by reducing drinking or stopping altogether. The client decides which is better: moderation or abstinence. The site advises: *The Alcohol Management program is for people with mild to moderate alcohol problems who want to eliminate the negative consequences of their drinking. Alcohol Management is not for those who are severely dependent or alcoholic and require treatment approaches rather than educational ones.* This approach involves actual phone or in-person counseling sessions. The counselors all have master's degrees in social work or related mental health disciplines. The program is licensed by the State of Michigan Office of Substance Abuse Services. It involves a one-hour assessment, then four one-hour individual sessions or five two-hour group sessions or four 40-50-60 minute telephone sessions.

Alcohol Management also recommends a two- to three-week hiatus from drinking. The goal of this brief period of abstinence is to re-establish one's alcohol tolerance. The idea is that once you start drinking again, you re-learn how your body experiences alcohol.

Although I am not advocating that clients participate in this program, it is introduced here to reference another program geared towards controlled drinking rather than abstinence. It is mentioned, but clients may also decide to further investigate at home.

Some of the strategies developed by the Alcohol Management and Moderation Management approaches include the following:

- Delay drinking. Don't have anything alcoholic until you sit down to dinner.
- Quit drinking mixed drinks. Stick to wine or beer.
- Alternate alcoholic drinks with water or other nonalcoholic beverages; examples include nonalcoholic beers, "mocktails" (e.g., Virgin Marys), sparkling water or club soda with a slice of lime.
- Never drink alcoholic beverages when thirsty. Quench your thirst first with water.
- Don't drink alcohol after fasting.

And one of my own suggestions is to remember that sometimes your feeling on the way home from work that you are craving a drink is really a craving for food. So eat some healthy snacks before drinking.

In addition to the above-referenced techniques, I have also found it helpful to incorporate a neuro-linguistic programming approach, which allows clients to mentally rehearse via hypnotic suggestions being in situations in which they are about to drink. They are told:

> I want you to imagine looking at a giant movie screen … and you know that many TVs nowadays have a picture-in-picture feature. I want you to see yourself in the main picture, which includes most of the screen, in a social setting that involves drinking … Perhaps at a party, or a dinner with others who drink before or with dinner, or maybe you are in a bar with friends … and I want you to imagine the way you used to respond to such a situation, the way you used to respond, perhaps even imagine the beginning of intoxication … but then in a little insert in the lower right corner, see yourself the way you would like to be, saying "NO" after you have had your intended limit of drinks (assuming you are not driving – if driving, no more than one, preferably none), or sooner so that you can pace yourself and drink some later, perhaps drinking water instead … next I want you to imagine the little picture becoming larger and larger, brighter and brighter, the big picture, and the way you used to respond … becoming smaller and smaller, dimmer and dimmer … so at some point the little picture, the way you want things to be becomes the larger picture … the new, big picture the way you want to be, in control of your drinking, and now the picture of the way things used to be is a tiny insert in the upper left hand corner, and it is small and dim.

I typically repeat this process three times, with the suggestion that "three" is the "magic number" that will lock it into their subconscious mind.

As with the Abstinence Model, work is also done on investigating, through hypnotic regression, underlying self-defeating motives. The client is told, for example, while hypnotized:

> Since you consciously want to maintain a controlled approach to alcohol, but have been having trouble doing so, perhaps there is something going on at a subconscious level that causes you to self-sabotage. I am going to teach you a hypnoprojection technique to help you uncover these subconscious motives.

I then use the imagery of a blank screen, a projector, and a roll of film. I tell them that the film is a symbolic representation of their own subconscious mind, and by rewinding the film, we can look back into the past and review significant events that may have been early origins of the tendency to self-sabotage.

As noted in other places in this book, "stories" (metaphors) are given both in and out of hypnosis. Such stories provide an indirect communication and often assist the client in reframing. One example of an evocative little image is the concept that when one is drinking, the alcohol depresses the inhibitory centers of the brain, thus resulting in the cliché sometimes by people or about people who are intoxicated on alcohol being "10 feet tall and bulletproof." Because their usual inhibitions are repressed, they have a sense of power or of not caring about anything, which results in a temporary sense of empowerment. It is this sense of empowerment that might make the client seek a certain level of intoxication; thus the idea of controlled drinking, so as not to get to that point of imagined "freedom from inhibition."

## Relapse Prevention

First of all, the word "relapse" implies total failure and return to their previous condition. It may lead the client to think, "Well I blew it, so I might as well continue using for a while." I remind them that one of the clichés often heard in A.A. is, "Our goal is progress, not perfection." Therefore, they can use the words "mistake," "error," or "slip," instead of relapse. These words might be less ego-threatening than "relapse." Relapse can be a very tricky situation for alcoholics or heavy drinkers. After even a short period of sobriety the client may begin to think that they are out of the woods, so to speak. Both in the early stages of treatment and after the client reports at least short-term sobriety, stories/metaphors are used to reinforce their efforts. One story told in or out of hypnosis is as follows:

> A man came to see me with the following story: he had been a "very bad alcoholic for years." He said that he was so bad that it got to where he couldn't drive anymore because he no longer had a license or auto insurance, having wrecked so many cars. He said he finally saw the light and got involved with AA. He got so involved that he began to sponsor other alcoholics. He was sober for seven years. He was on the AA speaker circuit. Then the unthinkable happened. His wife got pneumonia and died

shortly after giving birth to their seventh child. He said, "Nothing could have made me believe that I would ever take another drink. But I didn't know my wife would die. I've been drinking ever since!"

The above story is one involving exceptional circumstances. More often than not, the situations or stimuli that trigger the person's habit to use their chosen substance are much less dramatic, sometimes almost reflexive. A story I tell such individuals involved an older woman who was a chronic alcoholic. She reported:

Whenever I try to quit and am sober for a few days, my husband sabotages me. He is a cab driver. He drinks very little. But sometimes when I am sober for a while, he will come home for dinner with a bottle of wine. He will say, "I just felt like having a little wine with my dinner." He will drink one glass, finish eating, and then go back out to work. I will, of course, finish the bottle of wine, then walk to the liquor store, buy a bottle of vodka, and be drunk for days. While I am drunk, I pretty much stay in the bedroom. He is very sweet, brings me meals in bed, has sex with me, and goes back to work.

I explained to her that he appeared to be sabotaging her in order to control her. I explained that when she is drunk, she is totally dependent on him. This state insures that she won't sober up and leave him … It was suggested that she get him involved in her treatment, so at least he would be held somewhat accountable … to the therapist, if not to anyone else, and perhaps would discontinue the sabotage.

## Uncovering

With alcoholics, problem drinkers, and the other addictions described in the following chapters, the "uncovering" technique is often an important aspect of the program. To give the client an example of the power of this technique, I tell the story about a girl whose problem had nothing to do with addictive behavior; rather, it had to do with self-esteem.

Years ago, when I was on rotation to do psychological testing at an adolescent psychiatric hospital, I was called to see a 16-year-old girl admitted to the unit. The nurse told me when I arrived: "This kid feels like she doesn't fit in, and she really doesn't. The other kids don't like her, and we don't like her." Well, they didn't actually admit that, but it was the impression I got ... But, I liked her. She was a pretty girl, but thought she was ugly, of course. A few days after completing the examination, I received a call from the Unit Nurse. She said: "Dr T, you are the only one who connected with this kid. Would you like to follow her on an outpatient basis when she is discharged?" I replied: "Yes, but since I'm there a couple of days a week anyway, how about if I start seeing her as an inpatient, then at my outpatient office after discharge?" The hospital staff agreed. In our first inpatient treatment session, I talked with her about this feeling of never fitting in. She admitted that she felt that way, but did not know from where it originated. It was just always there. I talked with her about hypnosis, if her mom agreed, but noted it was too noisy there, with kids making noise in the hallways, the overhead speakers, and so forth, but said we could do it when she came to my office. In our very first outpatient session, hypnosis was begun. She entered a hypnotic state easily. I had her imagine watching a movie of her life, and told her as I counted backwards from five to one, the film would rewind, and when we got to one, a picture would come into focus on the screen that would tell us about some very significant experience in her past related to the problems she had in the present with not fitting in. When I got to one, she told a story that had occurred when she was three years old. She said she had just gotten out of the bathtub, so she had no clothes on, and was playing on the floor with her dolls. Her mother entered the room and severely berated her ... she told her what a nasty, naughty little girl she was ... shame on you, NAKED! Tears were running down the child's face as she described this scene. I remember thinking, boy what a mean mother, but I'll bet that wasn't the first time something like that had occurred. So I told her that I was going to count backwards again, and this time when I got to one I wanted her to tell me about the very first experience in her life that might relate to why she always felt that she didn't fit in. She described an incident when she was an infant. She didn't know how old she was, but knew that she didn't know how to talk yet, but she could hear. She was in a baby crib, and she could hear her mother and her grandmother arguing in the next room. The grandmother was saying, "I told you that you should not have had that baby. Her father wouldn't marry you. There is no place for her in this world." At this point, she again cried profusely.

That was the insight part of the technique. Next, I wanted to re-program her thinking about these experiences. I said: "You know, it doesn't sound to me like you had a very nice grandmother. I know I surely don't like her. To say the least, she didn't seem to have the sensitivity or ability to love and accept you, and to cherish you the way you deserved. But what if you had the most wonderful grandmother in the world, one with all of the Christ-like (I don't do religious counseling, but I knew she was a Christian, so used it) qualities of love, and compassion, and empathy ... what if you had that kind of grandmother? What would she have said?" Her tears turned to a big smile, and she offered: "She would have said, 'what a beautiful baby! I'm so glad we have her!'" To which I said: "And that is what most grandmothers would have said. Unfortunately, you were stuck with this mean-spirited grandmother who was incapable or unwilling to give you the love you deserve. But **that's not your fault!**"

"Now let's go back to when you were three years old, playing naked on the floor with your dolls. If you had the most wonderful mother in the world, one with all of those Christ-like qualities, or better yet, if you were the mom and it was your three-year-old daughter, what would you have said?" She responded: "I would have said: Honey, it's not good hygiene to play on the floor without any panties, so you can get dressed and play or you can get up in the bed and play." To which I asked: "You mean you wouldn't have told her she was a BAD GIRL?" She responded, "Of course not!" "Well, then, were you a bad girl? I asked." And she responded, "OF COURSE NOT!" Once again, the idea was reinforced that **it's not your fault!**

The client is then told:

She left that day like a different person. Now, not in all cases that we do such uncovering work are the results that dramatic, or achieved that quickly, but this case gives you an idea about how things that happened long ago might have some impact on your life in the present.

Uncovering/regression is just one among many strategies utilized to assist the client in learning to understand the origins of self-sabotaging or self-handicapping behavior.

Another story I sometimes tell involves an individual who went from being a child movie star to being a heroin addict to being a "born-again Christian." He then returned to his home town, went back to school, got a master's degree in counseling and became a substance abuse counselor. He told his story many times in open meetings. One of the statements he made was that he was an "addictive personality" in the truest sense. He said, "Even if I'm home watching a ball game and drinking a diet soda, I'll drink a whole six-pack of soda during that game." For such individuals, abstinence may be the only model!

The following stories impart little insights about relapse prevention. I tell them as a way to help clients understand some of their own feelings and vulnerabilities. I call the first story "The Road Home" and the second "The Prize Fighter."

### The Road Home

A fellow was on his way home after work on Friday. He had just gotten paid, cashed his check, and was walking home, only to be accosted by some thugs who mugged him and took all of his money. When he got to his home, his neighbor and friend, who was outside cutting the grass, saw that he was beaten and bruised and said, "Man, what happened to you?" The victim told his story. The friend said, "I'm sorry you had such a bad thing happen to you." The next Friday, the exact same scenario occurred. The neighbor again saw his buddy beaten and said, "Not again?" After the victim told his story, the neighbor advised: "I think you'd better take a different route home!" After several weeks passed, during which he did take a different way home, another Friday came and he arrived home beaten up and mugged. He announced to his neighbor, "It happened again!" The neighbor responded, "But I thought you were taking a different way home?" The man answered: "I FORGOT!" And this is often what happens after a brief period of sobriety. We forget how distressed we were when we entered treatment and backslide into old maladaptive behaviors.

### The Prize Fighter

Even a pretty good boxer might eventually get to a point where he seems to have lost enough of his skills that the young talents are beating up on him. He decides it is time to hang up the gloves. He retires. Time passes. But then his body begins to recover from the beatings. He starts working out again. Finally, he begins to think "I'm stronger than ever. I'm in great shape. I can make a comeback!" So his agent or trainer or promoter gets him some fairly easy fights with "nobodies," and he wins! He then feels ready to take on the young studs again. It is not long until he gets his block knocked off. He retires again, hopefully, for the last time, but some have attempted several comebacks before they realize, "I just can't do it anymore."

This metaphor seems to be especially relevant for individuals who have a history of drinking problems, followed by periods of sobriety, followed by failed attempts at social drinking. Often times, these clients were successful in maintaining a moderate level of drinking for awhile; for example, having only a couple of glasses of wine when out to dinner. Then they crash and burn, not stopping at two, but perhaps drinking many more until severely intoxicated and getting into trouble.

The following is a story I often tell clients who apparently need (based on their failure at Moderation Management) to abstain from alcohol altogether, but hate the thought of never being able to drink again.

### Las Vegas High

A man told me that he was actively participating in AA, was using the self-hypnosis techniques I was teaching him, and was doing fine with the idea of one day at a time, but hated the thought of "missing out" on some of the really good times he had had that involved heavy alcohol consumption. When I asked for an example, he said: "Okay, I can think of one. I was in Las Vegas on a junket. My buddy's girlfriend brought her best friend with her. We wound up hooking up. One morning, in the wee hours, I was at a blackjack table. I was winning about $3000, drinking, smoking a cigar, and this beautiful blond was sitting like halfway between my legs at the table. I decided to quit while ahead *(obviously he was able to be a controlled gambler when there was incentive),* picked up my chips, and the blond and I went to my room. We ordered room service and at daybreak we were sitting in the Jacuzzi, drinking Dom Perignon, eating strawberries, and then had great sex. I hate to think I'd never to be able to do that again!" I responded: "Well, that sounds like a very fun and exciting night, but now how many times has that happened compared to how many times you saw the blue lights and were arrested for DUI, or woke up both sick and broke, or screwed up relationships when drinking?" Of course, I already knew from our interviews the answers to these questions. He promptly came back with: "Wow! You're right. That was just *once*! I have had many more negative consequences from drinking."

In addition to the stories, I employ other techniques. I often draw a diagram that I saw a drug counselor at one of the hospitals at which I consulted draw in one of his group sessions.

HEALTHY   &longleftrightarrow;   HEALTHY
SICK   &longleftrightarrow;   SICK

The counselor went on to describe how healthy people attract healthy people and sick people attract sick people. And never do the two meet. This is especially important for clients who become sober and now have to deal with different and problematic interpersonal dynamics with their significant other. I explain:

> Often, the addiction becomes a focus of difficulty between the couple. One partner might say, "Everything would be fine if he would just stop drinking (or drugging, or gambling)." But then the person stops the problem behavior and the mate still doesn't like him. The focus on the addiction was just a smokescreen masking deeper incompatibilities. Or, there may be times when you give up the problem behavior and find that you can't stand your mate. Maybe while "using," you always felt guilty or somehow deficient, thus asking yourself, "Who am I to think I deserve better?" But when you are clean and sober, you might begin to feel that perhaps you do deserve better. Perhaps it was your significant other's "sickness" that allowed the two of you to remain together even while you were using. And now clean and sober, the terrain has changed.

Such discussions often help the client realize the unseen dynamics that are likely in play that might cause setbacks if they remain out of awareness.

When there is a patient who has a history of blackouts, I remind them of a harsh potential reality often overlooked:

> One of the worst things about drinking to the point of not remembering the events of the past evening is your inability to defend yourself. You could literally be accused of murder and not remember enough to defend yourself. While I have never worked with anyone accused of murder during a state of intoxication, I have seen clients who were accused of things like wife beating and of child molestation. At least if you are sober, whether through abstinence or moderate drinking, you can remember the events of the prior evening well enough to defend yourself against possible false allegations.

In summary, some hypnotherapeutic approaches to abstinence and controlled drinking are presented in this chapter. At the center is the hypnotic reinforcement of the 12 Steps of AA as well as brief metaphors/stories to help the client gain and maintain sobriety.

# Chapter Three

# Focus on Drug Abuse and Addiction

As noted in the Introduction, there has not been a lot published in the literature regarding the use of hypnosis or hypnotherapy with this clientele. In the syllabus on hypnosis I received at my very first ASCH conference in 1978, there was only one reference (LaScola, 1973).

In this chapter, I will present my experiences and techniques with the utilization of hypnosis in treating drug users and describe a number of techniques, metaphors and scripts.

As described in Chapter 1, in my early experiences with hypnotherapeutic treatment, a young woman with back pain was referred. She told me that her pain management specialist had said that he had done all he could for her, but perhaps someone who did hypnosis could help. We planned a course of hypnotherapy. It was first explained that nobody in our office thought that the pain was all in her head; rather, the intent would be to help her learn to de-stress and relax, which would help her to learn to reduce the level of her subjective pain. At the end of the very first session, however, when asked, "How do you feel?" She responded, "Damn, that was better than drugs!" It was learned that she and her husband, in their earlier years of dating and marriage, used to get high quite often. Their drugs of choice were Quaaludes (a popular prescription drug then, now banned) and marijuana (primarily downers/relaxants). She said they still smoked "weed" regularly. This incident led to an important realization; if this patient responded in this way, perhaps others, including drug abusers and addicts, could be convinced that hypnosis was a "natural" way to at least relax, if not get high. This idea seemed especially relevant for individuals who were using drugs to "self-medicate" for anxiety issues.

The techniques developed to utilize with this population are very similar to those used with alcoholics and problem drinkers. With drug abuse and addiction, however, the goal is always abstinence, not moderation. The techniques, then, can be incorporated from Chapter 2, which is accomplished by substituting the particular drug or drugs of choice for alcohol in all of the hypnotic suggestions. Just as alcoholics are encouraged to attend a pre-planned number of Alcoholics Anonymous (AA) meetings per week, the drug user is strongly encouraged to attend Narcotics Anonymous (NA) meetings. However, be forewarned that in my experience, drug users are more resistant to 12-Step programs because of the legal implications of many drugs of abuse. Therefore, in my work going to meetings is not mandatory; rather, I offer it as an adjunct.

As discussed in Chapter 2, as with alcoholics and problem drinkers, I believe that despite our dislike of managed care, programs should be tailor-made for the individual client. All drug addicts are not created equal. For example, the couple who occasionally smoked a little pot in their garage so that their adolescent daughter wouldn't know (she did, of course) is quite different than the prescription drug abuser/addict, who in turn may be quite different from the crack cocaine addict. Given this fact, individualized treatment plans make much more sense than a standard 30-day residential treatment plan.

I had some experience in the 1970s in which it was determined that many of the drug abusers seen at a rural community mental health center were "white, middle-aged, middle-class, female pill-poppers." In fact, this was the initial title of the paper, which was eventually published with a shorter title (Williams & Tramontana, 1975). At this point, there may be a more chronic and pervasive problem with prescription drug usage, especially painkillers, than with illicit drugs. The patient addicted to painkillers may be much "sicker" than someone who occasionally snorts cocaine at a party. On the other hand, I once had a patient with a "created identity" who made a very significant statement regarding recreational cocaine usage. His story was that he was in the "program" because he had been a state's witness against some drug smugglers, and he himself had had a very expensive cocaine addiction.

I mentioned to him once that I knew some people who claimed that they snorted cocaine recreationally. He responded: "Doc, anybody who can still use cocaine recreationally just hasn't been using it long enough yet!"

Early on in the sessions with drug addicts, as with alcoholics, we discuss the health risks of addictions. Prescription drug abusers typically already have associations with physicians (often several, unfortunately). I recommend that they have a physical examination if it has been more than 12 months since their last one. If they say they do not have a Primary Care Physician (PCP), I will typically refer them to one in their community. Although they are told that I am going to treat them psychologically/hypnotically, I believe in a holistic approach. I expect them to get a physical examination and to sign release forms that allow for the PCP and me to communicate regarding the patient's treatment.

I typically share various stories with them (in or out of hypnosis). One such story is presented by Larsen (1984) in his book entitled *Stage II Recovery: Life Beyond Addiction*. He talked about how while lecturing to a group of drug addicts, there was one individual in the room who had never spoken a single word in group. The speaker was describing to the group how life involves so many choices. He used the analogy of driving a bus. He explained that if you are driving a bus, and you come to an intersection, you have a number of choices available. You can go straight, turn left, turn right, refuse to move, or even do a U-turn and go back the other way. Suddenly, as if a light bulb went off, the patient who had never said anything before blurted out: "I finally understand. My problem is that for all of these years I have had a 'junkie' driving my bus!"

Next, patients might be told about the anti-drug ad put out by the National Institute of Drug Abuse that used to be in the Las Vegas airport. There was a picture that showed a pile of white powder, a razorblade, and a straw. The words "FAKE FUN" were spelled out in white powder. Next, it is pointed out that individuals who use drugs to "get high" or "have fun" are actually using an artificial stimulus and that this type of fun is not the same as skiing down a mountain slope, watching your children playing and laughing, laughing with friends and loved ones, etc.

When the drug use patterns have an obvious self-destructive bent, which they often do, additional attention is given in sessions (both in and out of hypnosis) to the subject of self-sabotage, We might discuss Pieper and Pieper's (2003) book entitled *Addicted to Unhappiness* or Carolyn Myss' (2002) archetypes, one of which is "Saboteur." Many times, individuals who are high-functioning tend to describe how just when everything seems like it is going well for them, they will do something to screw up. Such individuals are often not consciously aware of what might trigger their self-destructive tendencies. In such cases, hypnotic regression might be employed to help them uncover the origins of this maladaptive behavior. After a person is in a hypnotic state, they might be told, for example:

> I want you to imagine being back in that safe room we described in one of our previous sessions ... relaxing comfortably ... and on one wall of that room is a giant movie screen ... and a projector, and a reel of film (or perhaps to be more current, a giant TV screen and a DVD player) ... and this film is all about your life ... everything you have ever experienced is stored there ... in fact, the film is a symbolic representation of your own subconscious mind ... your subconscious knows everything about you ... everything you have ever seen, heard, felt, thought ... it is all there, and not only does your subconscious know everything about you, it knows what we need to know to help you with the problems for which you are seeing me ... I am going to count backwards from 5 to 1, and as I count, I want you to imagine the film rewinding, and when we get to 1, imagine a picture coming onto the screen, and that picture will tell us about some very important experience in your past related to the issues we are dealing with in the present ... the self-sabotage.

I typically start with "some very important experience" (less threatening to remember), then work toward "the most important experience" (more threatening to remember).

Another technique sometimes employed with drug patients is a takeoff on the control room metaphor for pain patients. My control room metaphor is a synthesis of Garver's (1990, p. 61) control switch visualization with pain patients and Hammond's (1990, pp. 354–355) master control room technique used with patients with sexual dysfunction. The patient is told:

> I want you to imagine that you can go into a place in your own brain … perhaps if you've ever been to Disney World or is it Universal Studios, there was a ride in which you were in like a spaceship and you were projected inside the human body to see the heart, lungs, etc. Let's suppose you could be projected inside your own brain. Your brain is the control center, much like the NASA Space Center that we see in all the space movies. The astronauts are always communicating with Houston. So imagine you can go inside this control center … in your brain. The brain is, in fact, your control center … imagine you come upon a lot of technical instruments … monitors, gauges, controls, and switches. And you see a monitor on the left … that has a gauge for tension or anxiety … and just to the right, one for calm and relaxation … and let's imagine that at first, the level on the left gauge … tension or stress, is a 9 on a 10-point scale … and the one on the right, the relaxation scale … is a 1 … Imagine that you can then begin to adjust the levels … there are knobs, like rheostats … and as you turn up the relaxation gauge from a 1 to a 2, with your right hand, you turn the tension/stress gauge down to an 8 with your left hand … next, you turn the relaxation gauge up to a 3 … and simultaneously turn the tension gauge down to a 7 … you continue … turning the relaxation gauge up to a 4, but as you are about to turn the tension gauge down to a 6, you notice a very interesting phenomenon … that knob seems to be turning by itself, automatically … and this is understandable, because tension and relaxation are incompatible responses. They are what we call mutually exclusive. You can't be tense when you're relaxed … and you can't be relaxed when you're tense … and so you interestedly proceed ahead … you turn the relaxation control up to a 5 and the tension automatically reduces to a 5 … now excited, you continue the process … you turn the relaxation up to a 6 and tension goes down to a 4 … then to a 7 and a 3 … etc. You might take them all the way to a 9 and 1, as a perfect 10–0 might be unrealistic.

This method seems to be very helpful for teaching clients a natural way to decrease levels of tension, stress, and anxiety. If the drug of choice is painkillers, one might have three gauges, two on the left (one each for pain and tension) and one on the right for relaxation. In that case, it is a similar approach to that above, except both the pain and tension gauges are lowered as relaxation is increased.

The phenomenon through which people develop an excuse for failure is described to clients. They are told (again, in or out of hypnosis) about the example of the college student who says: "I could have passed that exam, had I really studied, but I went out drinking with my buddies instead, and I flunked the test." The interpretation is that this may be less ego-challenging than to say: "I studied to the best of my ability, and I still flunked." So perhaps some individuals self-sabotage with drugs to "excuse" their lack of success or accomplishment, or their fear of failure (and/or fear of success?).

As with alcoholics, subsequent sessions are spent discussing progress, pitfalls, and issues of daily living, and then some work is done on the Steps, again, especially Steps 1 through 3. With severe drug abuse, a great deal of time is spent with uncovering the psychological reasons that the individual is self-sabotaging with substances.

In addition, the covert sensitization techniques (Cautela,1966) that are described in Chapter 4 with a gambling addict and in Chapter 5 with smokers, and the collapsing anchors technique (Zimberoff,1999) used with smoking (Chapter 5) are sometimes utilized.

Also of concern with drug abusers are cross-addictions. Cross-addictions concerns are why the traditional inpatient treatment programs recommend that drug users not drink, even if alcohol was not their drug of choice. Likewise, they recommend that alcoholics not smoke marijuana or go to casinos. It is explained to the drug using client that even if they had the best intentions not to use drugs, and drinking had never been a significant problem, a few drinks in an evening might weaken their self-resolve. Cross-addictions can complicate treatment in many ways. The mislabeling of the drug of choice, for example, can send attempts to plan treatment down the wrong road. Someone who uses both alcohol and cocaine might identify cocaine as their drug of choice only to find out that they are using cocaine to keep them up so that they can drink more for a longer period of time. In this case, the misidentification masks the reality of the situation.

Also discussed, both in and out of hypnosis, are the traditional alcohol and drug treatment clichés about having to change one's playgrounds and playmates (i.e., avoiding those people and places that might make the patient more susceptible to relapse). One story regarding this issue, which is given either in or out of hypnosis, is as follows:

> A client who described a situation in which he felt he was using cocaine (snorting) recreationally realized that the frequency and duration of his using was increasing. He came to see me and was highly motivated to quit using. He did fine for a few weeks. Then a friend with whom he used to "party" knocked on his back door at 3:00 am. He went to the door, very perturbed, looked out the window and shouted "What?" The friend, who was standing there with a girlfriend, opened up his hand, and flashed a gram of coke ... the client immediately opened the door and "graciously" welcomed his drug-bearing friend. This brief anecdote gives credence to the cliché frequently used by drug counselors; that is, you have to change your playgrounds and playmates.

Another story I often tell is as follows:

> When I was Director of the Regional Mental Health Center in Oxford, MS in the 70s, the University of Mississippi had legal marijuana growing fields for research purposes. A psychopharmacology professor from the University gave a presentation to our staff regarding the fact that their studies showed that marijuana was less dangerous than alcohol. He said they had research subjects do a number of field tests either after drinking or after smoking marijuana. After drinking, they tended to overestimate their motor skills. After smoking, however, they would say, "Man, I can't do that" (e.g., walk a straight line), but then do it perfectly.

Then I add the kicker:

> Shortly after I heard his talk, I worked with a patient who told me about how he used to go home for lunch daily, smoke a joint, eat, then go back to work ... one day, however, he returned to his work site and proceeded to saw off a finger with an electric saw!

This kicker, albeit anecdotal, may shed doubt on the statement often made by marijuana smokers that "smoking pot is safe."

Another technique involves what I refer to as a "problem-solving approach." The patient is introduced to a technique that I refer to as "Space Travel Meditation." The person is told to imagine that they are going to take a trip, and that travel is educational. It is emphasized that people who are well-traveled are often considered to be very wise, and, in fact, that is why schools take children on field trips, so they can be exposed to more of the world and how it works. I proceed:

> So I want you to imagine that we are going to take a fantasy trip into outer space ... first, I want you to imagine looking at your home, from ground level, and nod when you have that image in mind ... next, imagine looking down on your home from above, as you might see it from a helicopter or hot air balloon ... things look different looking down from above ... if you have ever been on the roof of your home, you remember how things look different from that vantage point ...
>
> Now you are so high you can see the entire area in which you live, as you might see it from a small plane ... and now the whole city as you might see it from a jet plane ... and now the entire region of the country, as you might see it from a spaceship or satellite of some sort ... getting higher ... you now see the entire continent ... and finally the whole of planet Earth ... until you are in outer space.

Then:

> Now I want you to imagine that on your journey you are going to visit somewhere in outer space. It could be another planet, or maybe a star ... the only restriction is that it will be only some place that is positive, or at least, neutral ... no places that are negative, evil, or scary ... and at least at one of your stops, you are going to meet an all-wise being ... he or she or it ... can be human-like, or it can be very different, but imagine this being has all the wisdom of the universe ... all of the wisdom of the cosmos available and is willing to share that wisdom with you ... so all you need to do is ask the questions, and the answers will come ... and most people will ask questions about issues for which they are seeing me. For example: What is this problem with my drug usage all about ... the next obvious question would then be, so what do I need to do differently? ... I'm going to remain quiet for a few minutes while you continue your journey, after which time I'll ask if you are ready for me to rejoin you ... then, I'll ask you to talk to me and tell me where you went ... who you met, what questions you asked, and what answers came to you.

After three of four minutes, I then rejoin the patient and while they are still in a hypnotic state, I ask the person to describe the experience. Important insights are often reported from this journey.

Later I explain that we all have much more wisdom, often in our unconscious or subconscious mind, than we realize. That is why, for example, when we attend a continuing education conference to learn something new, we might leave thinking, "I knew that!" And the answer is that we often know much more than we realize that we know. So this Space Travel Meditation is a technique to channel information from our own unconscious minds, through the all-wise being, back to our conscious minds.

In my work with drug abusers, I have found that resentments are as much or more of an important factor with this group than with alcoholics. So, just as I explain in Chapter 2 in working with alcoholics about the difficulty with Step 9, making amends, I find it equally important to explore the drug addicted person's anger and resentments.

In summary, using as many techniques as possible to investigate self-defeating possibilities should be given priority. A number of techniques, metaphors, and scripts should be discussed, but some time must also be devoted to helping clients discover their own techniques for discovering their self-sabotage motives. Again, much of the information presented in the previous chapter on alcohol abuse is relevant to drug abuse and can be used effectively in treatment with drug abusers. The scripts, metaphors/stories can be adapted simply by substituting the drug of choice or by simply giving a generic suggestion regarding "substances."

# Chapter Four

# *Focus on Gambling Addiction*

I have found even less in the literature regarding hypnothera-peutic techniques for pathological gambling than for alcoholics and drug abusers. Recently there was a case study presented by Chapman (2008) in which he worked with a client whose pre-senting problem included several issues, only one of which was compulsive gambling (on-line poker). In the fifth of five planned sessions, gambling was addressed. A combination of clinical hyp-nosis and cognitive behavior therapy was used. The author of that study reported that the client realized that his statement that, "I always have a chance at winning if I am playing" was not evi-dence based. In fact, he admitted that he seldom won. The client reportedly decided to give his personal computer to his brother and to only use his office computer for business.

In my own work, I use many of the same basic techniques for gambling addiction as for alcoholism and drug addiction; how-ever, there are some additional approaches that have specific relevance for this population. Keep in mind that the scripts for alcoholics presented in Chapter 2 regarding hypnotically reinforc-ing the 12-Step approach should be reviewed.

Not all gamblers are pathological gamblers, no more than all drinkers are alcoholics or even problem drinkers. The groups of elderly people who take the bus to the casino once a month are likely not gambling pathologically. Likewise, there are many peo-ple who find casinos, horse races, friendly poker games, bingo, or betting on sports events quite entertaining. Clients are typically told that the behavior is only pathological if it is controlling you instead of you controlling it. The clients are given a question-naire, which includes items similar to those given to my smoking cessation patients (see next chapter) and similar to items on the MAST (Michigan Alcohol Screening Test).

*Betting Questionnaire*

1.  At what age did you make your first bet?

2.  Where were you/on what were you betting?

3.  Did you win that bet?

4.  Has there been a progression in the amounts bet?

5.  Have you ever lied to anyone important to you about the extent of your gambling?

6.  Have you ever thought you were gambling too much?

7.  Have you had arguments/conflicts with others about your gambling?

8.  Do you ever feel guilty about gambling?

9.  Have you tried to quit or cut back? If so, what happened?

10. What is your goal for this treatment?

## *Early Experiences*

My primary office for many years was on the Mississippi Gulf Coast, an area where there were, before Hurricane Katrina, many dockside casinos. Since Katrina, they are being re-built as land-based casinos. Even before casinos existed in the area, a patient presented to me with a gambling addiction. He indicated that he gambled on everything – sports through local bookies (nowadays many people bet via the internet with off-shore casinos), and poker games – but his primary addiction was the dog track in Mobile, Alabama. This individual (a police officer) admitted many characteristics thought to be common in gambling addicts, including embezzling money from his job, lying about his activities, and hocking his wife's jewelry with the intent of winning and then buying it back. What was interesting and unusual, however, was that he said he never, ever won, not even on one occasion. The literature suggests that gamblers who win their very first wagers are highly likely to become addicted. But this guy never won! His pattern is very inconsistent with what will be described below regarding intermittent reinforcement. This fact made understanding his behavioral patterns even more complicated than usual. Diagnostically, his behavior never being reinforced might suggest it more maladaptive than is typical.

Basically, the program developed for him involved covert sensitization (Cautela, 1966). However, the difference from Cautela's approach was that the suggestions were presented hypnotically. The client was told to imagine being at the dog track, reading the past performances chart, and making his betting choice or choices. Then he'd go up to the window, and as soon as he told the attendant his choice, he would begin to feel nauseated. This would be carried so far as to having him vomit all over the ticket given to him by the attendant, all over the countertop, himself, and so forth. After leaving the ticket window and going to the men's room to clean up, he felt very relieved being away from the gambling and the vomit. The client reported significant improvement following just a few hypnotic sessions. It is noteworthy that covert sensitization is not recommended for someone who may also be bulimic.

My experience with gambling addicts is that it is an addiction almost as serious as crack cocaine addiction in the degree of deviousness involved in it. The gambling addicts I have worked with will steal, lie, and cheat in order to fund their addiction.

I remember all the way back to undergraduate years (Psychology 101) the descriptions of operant conditioning and the various reinforcement schedules. Behavior that was randomly reinforced was always the hardest to extinguish. It seems as though I remember Skinner talking about training animals to "gamble" based on intermittent reinforcement schedules. And for years, when counseling parents regarding child management, I talked about the importance of consistency. I described their sometimes giving in immediately and sometimes after several nags or "begs" from the child as a variable ratio schedule akin to what I referred to as "slot machine theory." That is, "If I keep trying, sooner or later I'll hit the jackpot!" For most gambling addicts, it appears that this variable ratio schedule may serve to strengthen the addiction. In other words, other than the patient mentioned above, for most people, losing every time would extinguish the behavior. The logical response would likely be: "This machine/game/casino/ lifestyle isn't working anymore." But it is more probable that the gambler will receive intermittent reinforcement, thus creating the condition for continuing the addiction. In treatment, just as with alcoholics and drug addicts, some time is dedicated to describing to the client the "acting-out cycle."

## *Current Techniques*

I believe that it is important for the client who wants hypnosis to quit gambling to know that the therapist is somewhat knowledgeable about gambling. Being a somewhat experienced albeit not pathological casino blackjack player and having spent some time at horse tracks, I have compiled the following brief list of gambling "lingo":

- *Bankroll*: The amount of money the player takes with him to the casino or other gambling venue. This amount is often the amount the gambler has to "play with." Professional gamblers, who gamble for a living, as opposed to pathological gamblers, will typically not lose more than their bankroll in one gambling session. In other words, they will not access lines of credit, ATM machines, or cash checks. Rather, they are likely to accept the fact that it is just "not their day," and leave until they feel the time is right for their fortunes to be reversed.

- *Lines of Credit:* Casinos will often give *high rollers* a line of credit (often $10,000 or multiples of that amount) based on their credit history. Typically, the gambler will have had to provide the casino with bank account information. If the player does not settle up their *markers* before leaving the casino or by some agreed-upon timetable, the casino can collect on that marker directly from the player's bank account.

- *Markers:* A marker is a paper with carbonized copies for the player and the *house,* which serves as a bank draft should the player not settle-up with the casino before leaving or by the pre-arranged date.

- *House:* The *gambling facility.* Might be a casino, website, video poker hall, racetrack, etc.

- *High-rollers:* This term is somewhat self-explanatory. It typically refers to someone who has a lot of money and gambles large sums.

- *Whales:* As opposed to *high-rollers*, who may win or lose large sums, *whales* typically only lose, dumping large sums of money into the house coffers.

- *Comps:* Casinos use many different promotional techniques to attract players. They send mail-outs with coupons for free meals, match-play chips, and raffle away cars to people who are playing at the time. But *comps* are the greatest means of attracting players. Comps refer to free rooms, food, beverages, and sometimes the player's airfare. Someone who is being "comped" room, food, and beverages, for example, is said to be *RFB (Room, Food and Beverage).* It should be noted that "comps" are not just given to losers. It is based on the players amount of time playing and their average bet (which is monitored either by pit bosses for the table games or players club cards inserted into the machines). If a player is a big winner, the casino certainly wants them to come back and give the house a chance to get their money back.

I spend some time educating gambling addicts regarding these facts; that is, how the gambling behavior has been reinforced, and why it has continued. I also throw in some mathematical concepts such as the "law of large numbers." This concept basically means that if they are playing a game in which the "house" has even a slight percentage edge (which they all do), they will eventually lose. Therefore, even if players win some of the time, if they play long enough the house will eventually beat them. I also talk with them about why the "house" (assuming they are casino gamblers) likes for them to win "sometimes." If no one ever won, the behavior might extinguish quickly. So even for someone who wins, the casino might provide "comps" in the form of free room, food, beverages, shows, air fare, because the owners know that the person who returns often enough will, sooner or later, lose and will likely spend lots of money trying to regain that high that came from winning.

I talk with them about how much of probability statistics was developed using gambling models, and how the casinos are quite aware of the statistics for their games.

I also discuss "the gambler's fallacy," which I came across many years ago. Basically, it states that if the gambler is winning, they say, "Well, why stop now. Now I'm playing with their money." If losing, they say, "I can't stop now, I need to recoup my losses." If breaking even, they say, "Why quit now? I didn't come here to break even!" So in all three scenarios, the gambler will keep playing, much to the house's delight!

Most often, cities that have casinos have billboards that advertise help lines for problem gamblers. In Baton Rouge, LA, the numbers are 1-800-770-STOP and 1-800-522-4700. When an individual calls one of these lines, they are asked if they have a problem with gambling and want help with it. People are typically referred to Gamblers Anonymous 12-Step programs in the area and/or counseling programs.

Gamblers, however, in my experience, are in some ways different from alcoholics or drug addicts when it comes to the 12-Step programs. For example, one patient came in for hypnosis to help prevent relapse. He claimed to be "clean" for a significant length of time. He reported that he had originated a local Gamblers Anonymous group. Prior to our hypnotic work, he indicated that he also had a lot of marital difficulties because of his history of gambling and that his wife would like to come in for conjoint sessions. After a few of these conjoint sessions, and before hypnotic work was ever begun, I got quite a surprise. While on the escalator of a casino heading to the casino restaurant to partake in their Alaskan King Crab special, I spotted this client at a Blackjack table near the escalator. The client saw me as well. He came alone to the next session. He indicated that he wanted to make sure that our relationship was totally confidential and that his wife would never be told of that situation. I questioned him about whether while he was actively participating and even leading meetings of his Gamblers Anonymous group, he had ever shared that he "slipped." He said that he had not and added, "Look Doc, everybody in GA meetings still gambles!" When questioned about how this could be, he said that he knew this because he would often see other group members when he was at the casinos.

The only explanation that seemed plausible was that GA is much newer than AA and NA, and in this local area perhaps there wasn't a whole lot of sobriety in those meetings. The "old timers" in AA/NA often provide a guiding influence to help the newcomers in their recovery. If there are no "old timers" in a particular group, the situation might be very different.

Another interesting case involved a woman whose aspiration was to become the women's world champion poker player. This was before we had all of the poker games on television (ESPN even treats it like it's a sport). This woman was very well-dressed and quite physically attractive. She owned her own business and presented with class and dignity; yet she informed me that she would often leave her business and home on a Saturday afternoon and head to a coast casino with her husband, who also liked to gamble. Within a few hours of being there, however, he would be ready to drive home. She would tell him to go on without her and that she would get a ride home later. Sometimes "later" was not until Tuesday. When questioned about whether she stayed in the casino hotel, she indicated that she never left the casino except to go to the ladies' room to freshen up – no baths, no changing of clothes, only quick meals from the snack bar. This woman was not really motivated to quit gambling and dropped out of treatment before it really began.

For clients who are motivated to change, however, change can occur. In working with gambling addiction, the techniques described in Chapters 2 and 3 for alcoholics and drug addicts are utilized. In Session 1, the first three steps of the 12-Step program are hypnotically suggested and reinforced. The difference, of course, is substituting gambling for alcohol or drugs. For example: *I came to admit that I am powerless over gambling, that gambling has made my life unmanageable.*

Session 2 with gambling addicts involves a similar approach to Session 2 with alcoholics and drug addicts, and subsequent sessions also follow the same course.

One hypnotic approach used with gamblers is a script described by Allen (2004) which he calls "Generic Habit Control" (pp. 49–52). This approach involves a number of colored doors, beginning with more pleasant colors and finally getting to a black door that opens to the part of you that encourages you to indulge in the problem behavior (gambling in this case) that you really want to break away from. It involves taking a position of strength, confronting that part that is the habit and threatening to banish the part unless it agrees now to cease the destructive behavior once and for all.

Cognitive-behavioral approaches, hypnotic regression regarding uncovering self-destructive patterns, the ideas regarding "addiction to unhappiness," and "self-sabotage" described in Chapter 3 are explored, both in and out of hypnosis. As the reader might expect, self-sabotage is a very important factor with pathological gamblers, who seem to continue their problematic behaviors regardless of the consequences (losing their homes, possessions, relationships, livelihood, and so forth).

As in the prior chapters, metaphors (story telling) occur both in and out of the hypnotic state. One story I often tell is:

> A former client who was seeing me for other issues, just happened to work as a Casino Host at a local casino. In one of our sessions, he was proudly relating to me how good he was at his job. He told me about the good care he took of his "good players." He mentioned, for example, that he had called an elderly couple who were good players, two weeks before

Thanksgiving. He told them: "Don't cook for Thanksgiving. If you already have a turkey, give it away or freeze it. I am going to send a limousine to your house on Thanksgiving morning with a complete Thanksgiving dinner, with all of the trimmings." He went on, "Everything from appetizers to dessert, including their favorite wine." When I finally interrupted him with the question: "What do you call good players," he responded, with a grin on his face, "People who lose a lot of money."

While casinos are famous for giving free drinks to players to "loosen" them up while at the casino, they also do many other things to entice people to come to the casino. They offer everything from special promotions that include "free" match-play chips or tokens, discounted rooms, automobile raffles in which you must play to be entered, to free rooms, food, and beverage (RFB) and even free airfares to high rollers. Many of the casino-type gambling addicts with whom I have worked are frequently "seduced" by what they see as "free" chances to win money. One female client, who was seeing me regarding "family problems," was in great denial about her gambling problem. Family members, however, were quite aware of it. She told me on one occasion about how she and her mom just went and played their "match play" chips. I responded that a gambling addict going to play just their match play chips would be akin to giving alcoholics free drinks during happy hour!

Cognitive-behavioral techniques, with somewhat of an educational bent, often are helpful in this area.

In May, 2008, I had the good fortune of attending a workshop presented by Dr. Dabney Ewin sponsored by the New Orleans Society for Clinical Hypnosis entitled "Ideomotor signals for rapid hypnoanalysis." At the time that I signed up for this continuing education experience (Ewin, 2008), I assumed that learning more about his approach would be of benefit to me in working with psychosomatic illness, especially since I work at a pain management clinic one day each week. I came to realize, however, that I could adapt his techniques to my work with addictions, as well. To provide a brief summary, Ewin teaches his patients ideomotor signals: that is, raising the index finger signals "yes," the long (middle) finger signals "no," and the thumb signals "I'm not ready to deal with that" or "I don't want to answer, yet." In the workshop and book of similar title, he described "seven common causes" of psychosomatic disorders. These include conflict, organ language, motivation, past experience, identification, self-punishment, and suggestion. To simplify, the theory is that since the left brain controls verbal behavior, logical and analytical thinking, and so forth, when questioned while in a hypnotic state, the client may still try to analyze what might be the most logical answer. The right brain, on the other hand, controls nonverbal behavior, creativity, reflexive or instinctive responding, and, in general, emotions or feelings. So his questioning always involves the phrases "do you feel" or "do you sense" that you are being affected by ____? (for example, conflict). Kroger and Fezler (1976, p. 46) postulated that one cannot talk to the unconscious. Rather, they believe Cheek's ideomotor signaling technique acts like a projective technique and, as such, can elicit valuable information.

I had learned about ideomotor signaling many years ago, and used it at times, but not in hypnotic uncovering of the origins of psychogenic disorders. One difference from his approach is that I always give an "I don't know" signal (the "pinky" finger). I ask that the client only use this as a last resort, since this response may make it too easy for the client to avoid a "yes" or "no" signal. One observation that has always amused me is that when instructed to answer with their fingers, some clients would give a yes signal while nodding from side to side (a "no" response) or a "no" signal while nodding up and down.

A case in which ideomotor questioning proved beneficial is as follows: A 40-year-old African-American hairdresser who owned a salon presented to my office. She had two children, ages 15 and 17. The "reason for contacting this office" on her personal data sheet was "relief of gambling." She reported that she has a very nice income, but has been averaging a $6000/month loss on slot machines. She said that she sometimes wins, but will often lose from $3000 to $4000 per week. She noted that she hadn't hocked her jewelry or lost her possessions. Based on my calculations, I believed her average loss to more than $6000 per month.

When I did the muscle testing (described in Chapter 1) with her, she began to cry when I asked her to think about the most positive thing in her life. When questioned about what made her cry, she responded that she thought of her children, but immediately began to think that she is cheating them. She noted that they have an average lifestyle, but if not for the gambling she could do so much more for them.

The first hypnotic induction was done in my initial session with her, in order to help her relax and leave that first meeting with a sense of optimism that help was forthcoming. She came back one week later and reported that she had practiced the self-hypnotic techniques that I had taught her the previous week for the first three days, but then "got too busy at work." She reported that she had only gone to the casino one time during the past week, as compared to her usual pattern of three to four times per week. She proudly announced that she took only $300 with her, no check books or ATM cards, and when she lost the $300, she went home.

After teaching her the ideomotor signaling technique (Ewin & Eimer, 2006; Ewin, 2008), I asked:

> One of the things that causes symptoms is what we call conflict. A conflict occurs when a person wants to do one thing and feels he or she should do the opposite. It is as if you feel you are being pulled in two directions. Answer with your fingers. Do you feel or sense that your gambling problem is caused by conflict? *She lifted the yes finger. I then asked:* Would it be alright for you to tell me about it? *She responded: "The relationship I'm in. I am really indecisive about the relationship." When asked how gambling fits into this indecision, she indicated that going to the casino took her mind off of her questioning herself about whether to discontinue the relationship.*

> *I continued:* Organ language is another thing that can cause symptoms. Organ language refers to phrases in our everyday conversation that include negative mention of a body organ like "I feel like I have been stabbed in the back." *She responded with the "no" signal. I said:* Another thing that causes symptoms is motivation. A person can be motivated to have a symptom because it seems to solve some other problem; for example, a student who gets sick at exam time. Do you feel that you are motivated to have this problem? *She responded affirmatively. When queried, she gave a very similar answer to the one she gave for conflict, that is, the relationship questions.*

Next:

> Another possible cause of symptoms is past experience. An emotionally charged event may cause immediate onset of symptoms or sensitize you so that some other analogous event will activate the symptom. Do you sense or feel that your gambling problem started with a significant experience in your past? *She responded affirmatively. I then asked:* Would it be alright to go back and make a subconscious review of everything that was significant to you in this episode? *After she raised her index finger, I asked:* Did it happen before age 20? *Since she indicated that it had not happened before age 20, I moved forward in 5-year increments (If she had indicated that it was before age 20, I would have gone backwards in 5-year increments). She gave the "yes" response to before age 35.*

Then I asked:

> Is it alright to orient your mind to what happened between ages 30-35 that relates to the present problem with gambling? *Her response followed:* I felt that I needed some alone time. I didn't enjoy going to movies alone, but the casino was a place I could go alone but be in a large group of people at the same time. I was alone but not lonely. Then when the relationship started, I needed even more time alone.

I determined at this time that she might need relationship counseling more than anything else at present, but she may not be ready to make a change in this aspect of her life.

> Another possible cause of symptoms is what we call identification. Do you feel that you are identifying with someone who had the same or a similar symptom? *She gave an affirmative signal. When questioned further, she indicated that her biological father suffered from drug addiction. She stated:* I remember my mother helping my father. They were apart but were still friends. She helped him to find help. He was really strung out.

She gave the "no" signal to questioning regarding whether her gambling could be some kind of self-punishment or a response to a suggestion or imprint. She indicated that her gambling started when she was in her early twenties, and it was not until her thirties that it became a problem. In summary, ideomotor signaling helped me gain some insights about the psychodynamic causes of this client's pathological gambling. Her treatment remains in the early stages, with some progress and some retrogression, but this technique helped in developing insights and in formulating a treatment plan.

One approach that has *not* proven effective in my practice is to create a managed approach to gambling (as in the Moderation Management approach to drinking), although it was attempted with at least a couple of patients. The clients were instructed to read books about money management methods for gamblers. Such approaches to casino gambling theoretically would result in always leaving with a significant portion of winnings still intact, assuming they did get ahead. One patient reported that this approach was working for him. He was now a "controlled gambler." Then he came in for a session and reported that after having been up several hundred dollars, he quit while ahead, took the cash out to his truck and hid it under his seat. He then went back into the casino, had a few drinks at the bar, got bored, went back out to his truck, and the rest is history. He lost his winnings plus another thousand.

This example also brings up the issue of cross-addictions. As noted above, casinos are famous for giving their players "free" drinks. It is for this reason that traditional AA/NA-based rehab programs tell their patients they "can't go" to casinos and stay clean and sober.

One particularly difficult case I encountered was that of a very successful professional. He combined primarily smoking and gambling. The husband of another successful professional and father of two young athletes, he was a "closet smoker." His "closet," however, was apparently the truck-stop gambling parlors (video poker) in the next county. He would go and play video poker, smoke cigarettes, and drink one or two drinks (although alcohol did not seem to be a major factor in the behavior, because he might just as well do that at dinner with friends or even at home, and never to excess). So the gambling was a getaway, in the evening (several evenings per week), where he had the "freedom" to do things he didn't do at home.

After a significant number of sessions, with no apparent improvement, I was somewhat frustrated about which direction to take. The client was intelligent and seemed motivated, but nothing changed. Then the idea came to look at other psychological issues. Psychological testing ensued. It turned out that he scored quite high on depression, anxiety, and obsessive-compulsive tendencies. It became apparent that the psychological issues were primary, and the smoking and gambling appeared secondary. In retrospect, it became clear that his patterns were quite consistent with obsessive-compulsive behavior. At the time of this writing, he had been referred to a Medical Psychologist (Louisiana has a law whereby psychologists can obtain prescription privileges if they have a master's degree in clinical psychopharmacology and pass the necessary exams). Some of the newer medications seem to be quite helpful with OCD as well as symptoms of depression and anxiety. However, shortly thereafter he terminated therapy with me, although he continues to see the Medical Psychologist for medication management. I suspect that he continues to go to the video poker establishments.

Another technique frequently used with pathological gamblers is the Space Travel Meditation described in Chapter 3 with drug abusers.

In addition to the covert sensitization mentioned earlier in this chapter with the patient who frequented the dog track, an approach referred to as collapsing anchors, presented by Zimberoff (1999), is sometimes utilized. The client is given the following suggestions:

> Now begin to get in touch with the behavior that you would like to reduce or eliminate in your life … gambling … Now, I want you to open up the hand that is **not** your dominant hand … face the palm up toward the ceiling … and begin to bring up the urge to gamble in this hand … whether it involves poker chips, cards, sitting at a slot machine or video poker machine … now I'm going to count from one up to five … and that urge to gamble will become stronger … 1 … you feel the urge to gamble coming up now … 2 … it is getting stronger and stronger and stronger … the desire to gamble … 3 … feel that urge, that craving coming up even stronger … 4 … it's really coming up … and 5. How strong is that urge now from 0–10? Zero means no desire, 10 is the strongest. Talk to me

and tell me how strong it is now. ... *(wait for response)* ... Now bring your attention to your most dominant hand, the one you associate with your addictive behavior ... Turn that palm up and put into this hand, the most repulsive, gross thing you can imagine. Get in touch with whatever it is that really grosses you out. Perhaps you can see it ... notice the color and texture ... maybe it really looks gross to you ... Let's begin to bring up that most repulsive feeling ... 1 ... really increase that awful experience in your dominant hand ... 2 ... perhaps you can really smell it ... that odor is so strong! That gross disgusting smell is nearly making you sick, it is so disgusting ... 3 ... feel that slimy feeling ... using all your senses ... 4 ... the way it looks, smells, tastes, feels ... that feeling of revulsion is getting stronger and stronger ... 5 ... What number is it now from 0–10? Zero means no feelings of disgust, 10 means the most. Tell me how strong that feeling is ... *(wait for response)* ... Now, in a moment, I will count to three and on the count of three, you will clap your hands together and hold them there. This will totally collapse the original urge to gamble ... Okay ... 1 ... 2 ... 3 ... Clap! Hold your hands together now ... just begin to feel or see this association in your mind ... the minute your hands touch, the association may begin to develop deep within your subconscious mind ... the association with that craving becomes mixed with this most repulsive image in your mind ... You can't even stand to think about gambling any-more. You immediately begin to feel sick, nauseous, uncomfortable when gambling is even talked about and you have to leave the area ... you find yourself repulsed at the thought of it. Notice how that gross experience has collapsed the urge for that original behavior.

All of the techniques utilized with alcoholism and drug addiction can be modified to work with pathological gambling.

In summary, gambling addiction is quite complex and all issues related to the behavior need to be considered. In this chapter, use of techniques/scripts described in Chapters 2 and 3 with alcohol-ics and drug abusers are described with respect to how they can be adapted to use with pathological gamblers. There are also a number of stories (metaphors) that I use with gamblers, which are presented. The importance of investigating or uncovering the psy-chological motives involved in self-sabotage is also discussed.

# Chapter Five

# *Focus on Smoking Cessation*

This chapter focuses on the three-session smoking cessation program I employ, as well as various marketing techniques regarding selling the program as a "package."

As most readers are aware, cigarette smoking is said to be even more addictive than heroin, yet it is legal! As with alcohol and drugs, the first session for clients who wish to give up tobacco includes interviewing them about health concerns. If they have not had a recent physical examination, they are instructed to do so.

A hypnosis marketing seminar some 10 years ago (Yarnell, 1998) yielded a number of marketing/packaging techniques for use with this population of clients. The presenter was a hypnotist, quite a salesperson, and not certified in any mental health or medical area. He was one of the originators of the "Traveling Seminar" approaches to smoking and weight loss programs (i.e., group sessions in which the hypnotist reserves a meeting room at a local hotel and carries out his program). One of his books provided additional ideas (Yarnell, 1996). Although much of what I learned at that seminar was not usable for ethical reasons – for example, many of the marketing/advertising techniques involved an over-glamorization of the programs and were inconsistent with the ethical guidelines of psychologists regarding advertising – what did, in fact, prove to be of great utility was his approach of packaging sessions. Before this seminar, my approach was to see clients on a session-by-session basis, just as in other psychotherapy cases. After the seminar, however, smoking cessation programs were sold in a three-session package. Further, the smoking cessation client was told the usual hourly fee and that they would be expected to pay all three sessions in advance, in return for which there would be a 20% cash discount. This approach ensures the client's commitment to the three-session program, is more cost-effective for the client and helps the therapist's cash flow.

If the client balks at the idea of paying that much money "up front," they are given information regarding the average annual cost to someone who smokes one pack per day. I have been using the figure $2000, although this amount may need adjustment as the cost of cigarettes continues to increase and according to the region in which people live.

In the past, during slow times, I ran newspaper ads offering a free 20-minute consultation. During this preview session, I went over the smoking questionnaire provided, presented an overview of hypnosis, and then made the case for the scheduling (and paying for) their three sessions.

Some authors/treatment providers recommend a two-session approach. Hammond (1990) notes that research shows that there is approximately a 25% success rate with one session and 65% for four to five sessions. I have not kept data regarding success rates with the three-session approach, but based on feedback from clients, it is estimated that the success rate is quite high for those who are motivated to change and stick with the three sessions. If clients are engaged in treatment because someone else wants them to change, such as doctors or family, the success rate is low. I share this information with clients in the first session. They are also told that this approach involves much work on their part; that is, success will be hard to attain if they come in expecting me to fix them.

The typical three-session format is presented next.

## *Session 1*

I first have my assistant give the client a smoking questionnaire (see Appendix A) to fill out in the waiting room. This question-naire asks typical questions concerning how much the client smokes per day, at what age did they begin, previous attempts at quitting, whether or not parents smoked, do significant others smoke (especially in the same house), and so forth.

After a hypnotic state is elicited, followed by breathing exercises, then deepening techniques, the client is told about the practice effect (See Chapter 1, p. 12), the generalization effect (See Chapter 1, pp. 12–13), and trance ratification ensues (See Chapter 1, pp. 13–14).

## 1. Regression to first cigarette

> The next thing I want you to do … in that safe, comfortable room that you entered after your elevator descent … I want you to imagine that on one wall in that room is a giant movie screen … it covers almost the whole wall and there is a projector and a reel of film. This reel of film is all about your life … it's like a documentary of your life … and in just a moment I'm going to count backwards from 5 to 1 … and as I count, I want you to imagine the film rewinding … and as the film rewinds, we're going to go back into your past … and what we're looking for today is that very first experience with smoking … I believe you said it was at age ___ … and I'll ask you to imagine a picture coming onto the screen … coming into focus on the screen. Then I'll ask you to talk to me all about it … tell me where you are … how old you are, but especially everything about your body's reaction to that very first cigarette. Let's rewind the film now going back in time … 5 … rewinding … 4 … going back in time … 3 … seeking, searching … 2 … and 1 … all the way back to 1 … imagine a picture coming into focus. I want you to tell me what you see, hear, feel, sense, or know about that very first cigarette. You have that image? Okay … and how old are you … Tell me all about it. I am especially interested in knowing how your body reacted to that first cigarette.

### After they have told me about the first cigarette:

> Okay … alright I want you to relax and concentrate on what I'm saying … for most human beings … that very first experience with cigarettes, or maybe even the first few … is very negative … you see, the natural human instinct is to reject foreign substances … cigarettes, tobacco, nicotine … these are all foreign to the human body. Think about it … if you get a speck of dirt in your eyes, your eyes are probably going to tear up, automatically … you don't have to think about it … to rid your eye of the foreign particle … or even a puff of wind in your eye and you probably

will blink, automatically. If you've ever attempted to siphon gasoline … it seems more guys have that experience than gals … but if you attempted to siphon gasoline and accidentally swallowed some, you probably would have gagged and maybe even vomited. The body's natural instinct is to reject the poison … reject the foreign substance. So that's what happens with smoking … for most people, that very first cigarette causes them to experience some negative symptoms … bad taste, hot taste, burning, choking, coughing, nausea … you see … but, they condition themselves to take in the foreign substance for social reasons … to be grown up … to be in … to be cool … to be sophisticated. You know there was a time in our history when it WAS the sophisticated thing to do … all the actors and actresses smoked on screen. Even the sports celebrities at one time advertised for cigarette companies. It was the in thing to do. There was a time when a high percentage of everyone over 14 years old smoked cigarettes. Nowadays, it is not the in thing … a very small percentage of people smoke nowadays … now, fitness is in, wellness … you see people joining health clubs, taking aerobics classes, lifting weights, running, jogging, swimming, bicycling … companies have walking tracks … hospitals have walking tracks and jogging paths and so on. Fitness is in … wellness is in. You certainly don't need cigarettes to be grown up. You have children of your own who are almost grown (or you are X years old) … You don't need it to be "in" because it's no longer the "in thing." It's not the sophisticated thing. Now, smokers are made to go outdoors and in some places, it's against the law completely. Since there are no longer any social reasons to smoke, I suggest that from now on, anytime that you put a cigarette to your lips, or even think about smoking a cigarette, I want you to flash back to the very first experience, when you were ____, smoking with your____ … and remember very vividly … the bad taste, the nasty taste, the feeling like you were going to be sick … all of those negative experiences come very vividly into your mind anytime you think about smoking a cigarette.

## 2. Rebel against the tobacco industry

Now a second reason why people start smoking at a young age is rebelliousness. We think of the words teenage and rebellious as almost synonymous. But it's not just teenagers who rebel, adults are rebellious too … and that's why some people have trouble quitting smoking … its like "you can't make me quit" … "nobody can make me quit" … it's a control thing … Years ago, there was a cigarette ad, I think it might have been Lucky Strike, which showed a guy with a black eye and he was saying,

"I'd rather fight than switch." He was talking about the fact that he'd rather fight than switch brands ... but nowadays there are still people who are saying, "I'd rather fight than quit." If you really need a cause against which to rebel, I suggest that you rebel against the tobacco industry, which has made their billions and billions of dollars at the expense of our health. They have known for years that smoking can cause premature death ... early death ... and that it is addictive ... but denied it all the while. The movie, *The Insider*, a few years back, with Russell Crowe, was about the scientist who first came forward and admitted that at one point the tobacco industry doubled the nicotine content in cigarettes in order to get more people addicted to the product. And he also admitted that they knew it caused disease, all the while they denied it ... Rebel against the tobacco industry that uses subliminal advertising to sell their product. Think of the Virginia Slim model ... the Marlboro man, the rugged old cowboy who was in all the billboard and magazine ads. The Marlboro man died a number of years ago of emphysema ... true story ... he really did use the product. *[While younger clients might not identify with these examples, almost all of the clients who have come to me to quit smoking are old enough to remember these characters]* ... Rebel against the tobacco industry's use of this type of subliminal stimulation to seduce you to buy their product ... and have you associate smoking with beauty, sexuality, virility. You see, if they had truth in advertising, they'd show people with lip and mouth cancer, and people coughing and choking and hacking. They wouldn't sell much of their product that way ... rebel against the tobacco industry, and if you need a model for your rebelliousness, the best example I can think of is the case of Patrick J. Reynolds. Patrick Reynolds was heir-to-be to the Reynolds's tobacco fortune. His grandfather started Reynolds's tobacco ... his father later ran the company ... his uncle owned Reynolds's Aluminum. He watched his grandfather, father, uncle, and two aunts all die of illnesses related to that lifestyle ... they were all smokers ... So at the ripe age of 40, Patrick started the campaign for a smoke-free America. He was immediately disinherited by the family, but he did it anyway. If you need a model, use him as YOUR model to rebel against the tobacco industry.

# 3. Habit Change

Next, I want to talk to you about habit change ... and one of the things we know from the psychological research laboratories is that habits are learned in stimulus–response chains. So when one stimulus elicits a response, that response becomes a stimulus for the next response, and that one for the next and so on down the line. What we know from these research studies is that the easiest place to break the chain is at the first possible link. So with smoking, the chain might be something like this … perhaps the thought of smoking, which could come from one of your triggers … if you usually smoke at a certain time, or with a meal, or in your car, or after a meal, in the morning, or whenever … or maybe seeing someone else smoke … that might be the stimulus for reaching for the package. Once you have the package secured, that might be the stimulus for taking out a cigarette … and once you have the cigarette out … that's the stimulus for lighting up, taking a drag, inhaling, exhaling, you see … So the best possible way to break that chain would be DON'T BUY CIGARETTES … Don't have them on hand … don't have a supply … get rid of them … throw them away … give them to a person you don't like, you wouldn't want to give poison to a friend … Get rid of your cigarettes, don't buy them. It's just like the alcoholic whom we tell, "Don't have alcohol in your home, and don't go to bars" … maybe later in their sobriety, they can go to a bar and drink a soft drink … or even, I know some recovering alcoholics who have alcohol in their home for friends and relatives who drink … and they never touch it … But at first, we say, don't tempt yourself. Don't have it on hand, get rid of your cigarettes … throw them away … don't buy cigarettes … you might also get rid of your lighters and ashtrays. Take control of your environment. So even if you have the thought … the urge … you don't have the means.

## 4. The Words "Need" and "Try"

Next, I want to talk to you about two words. The first word I want to redefine in your vocabulary and the second we are going to delete totally from your vocabulary … at least with respect to smoking behavior. The first word is "need." What is a need? Well, we need oxygen to live … you can't go too many minutes without oxygen, I don't think. If you have oxygen, you can live for awhile without water … but you can't go too many days without water … You need food to live, but people have been known to go quite awhile without food as long as they have water. In extreme climates, you need shelter, especially in extreme cold, for example. See, these are life or death needs … everything else is want. So tell yourself its okay to smoke if I really need a cigarette. But have you ever known anybody to die from not smoking a cigarette?

The second word is the word "try." I want you to completely delete the word "try" from your vocabulary, at least with regards to your smoking behavior. "Try" is a cop-out word, which implies the possibility of failure. For example, I have a pen in my hand right now. If you were to ask me to hand you or lend you my pen, I would say sure, reach over and hand it to you. But if I said, "I'll try," it would imply the possibility that I might not be able to get it to you … the possibility of failure. It's actually a pretty wimpy word, when you think about it. So from now on, I want you to use only affirmative statements with regard to quitting smoking. I have quit. I am a nonsmoker. I no longer smoke … or I am in the process of quitting. I am becoming a nonsmoker … only affirmative statements.

## For those patients who note in their questionnaire that they have a concern about gaining weight, I also include the following suggestion:

You mentioned in your questionnaire that you are concerned that quitting smoking may lead to weight gain. There are at least three reasons of which I'm aware that many people gain weight when they quit smoking. First of all, nicotine is a stimulant, so when you stop taking in that stimulant, you are hungrier. Second is the habit of putting something into your mouth. Third, tobacco smoke and all the chemicals in tobacco dull the taste buds, so once you quit smoking, food tastes better … in order to deal with these three issues, I recommend the following: First of all, drink more water. *[Most cigarette smokers I see drink very little water. While we would not want them to overdose with water over the long haul, increased water intake can be helpful while overcoming the cravings to smoke,]* Drinking lots of water will help fill you up and make you less hungry. It also satisfies that need to put something into your mouth, in this case, something that is calorie free. To deal with the issue regarding the taste buds, I recommend that you practice eating the way a gourmet food taster would taste food, or a wine connoisseur would taste wine. For example, the wine taster holds the glass up to the light to check the clarity, swirls it around in the glass to build up the full aroma and bouquet … brings it close to their nose inviting the olfactory sense into play, inhales deeply, and only then takes a tiny sip of wine into the mouth, swishes it around and brings all the taste buds into play, and only then does the wine taster swallow the tiny sip of wine … and this wine taster can get more enjoyment from this tiny sip of wine, in this way, then if they chug-a-lugged a whole glass … Practice eating in this matter. For example, cut your food into very small bites, and put down your knife and fork after every bite or after every other bite. Really chew your food and get every bit of flavor out of each tiny bite. This helps to slow you down, which gives the nerves in the stomach time to transmit the message to the brain that you are full. If you eat fast, by the time your brain gets the message that you are full, you're typically already past full. So eat slowly, focusing on the quality of food rather than the quantity.

## 5. *Three Meditational Statements*

[These meditational statements are an adaptation of Spiegel and Spiegel's (1978) smoking control techniques.]

Next, I want you to meditate on three statements. The three meditational statements are as follows:

1. For my body, smoking cigarettes is a poison. *(If the person chews tobacco or smokes cigars or a pipe, the suggestion is modified to fit the particular type of tobacco and intake.)*

2. This is the only body that I have.

3. And number 3 is a logical conclusion from 1 and 2. Therefore, if I want to live a long and happy life, I must respect and protect my body by only putting things into my body which are beneficial.

Typically, these meditational statements are repeated at least three times, telling the patient,

"You can paraphrase these statements however you like, as long as you get across these three basic ideas: For my body, smoking cigarettes is a poison. This is the only body I have. Therefore, if I want to live a long and happy life, I must respect and protect my body by only putting things into my body which are beneficial." *[Spiegel & Spiegel (1978) said, "… by not smoking cigarettes." I prefer to use a more positive statement.]*

Then, I bring the patient out of the hypnotic state by counting forward, after which time I teach them the three-step self-hypnosis approach described in Chapter 1 (p. 16) to practice at home. The patient is told to utilize the self-hypnotic techniques a couple of times a day, to think about the three meditational statements several times a day, especially at those times that used to be the highest probability times for smoking, and during the self-hypnotic state, to review all the things that they learned during this first session.

Clients are also instructed to keep a Daily Smoking Diary. I recall a study (I believe unpublished) done while I was a graduate student at the University of Mississippi in the late 1960s, which, although it involved behavior modification and not hypnosis, continues to be relevant. The volunteer subjects were told to keep a record for two weeks (baseline period) before treatment was to begin. They were to keep a little index card inside the wrapping of their cigarette packages and make an entry prior to lighting up. All of the volunteer participants smoked less during the baseline period than they had indicated smoking before. Each subject reported that just having to stop to make the entry sometimes caused him/her to decide not to smoke at that time. This is what we currently refer to as "mindfulness."

## Session 2

At the beginning of Session 2, the client is interviewed regarding their progress between sessions. If the client has stopped smoking completely or, as is more often the case, has cut down their intake significantly, they are reinforced for this degree of progress. They are told that they are now going to learn additional techniques that will enable working toward total abstinence. If the client reports no change, I investigate with them possible reasons, such as lack of true motivation to cease smoking and the importance of their maximal effort. In other words, I remind the client that hypnosis is not a magical cure; rather, it is a way of helping them to bring mindfulness into this habitual behavior. I often tell clients about the above-referenced behavior modification study when I was in graduate school and the importance of "mindfulness." I say:

> You know, habit behaviors tend to be automatic; you don't think about whether you should smoke or not smoke; it becomes automatic, like driving a car. Nor do you think about the consequences of smoking behavior. So habit behaviors tend to be mindless. In psychology and in hypnotherapy we have only recently begun talking about the importance of mindfulness. In places like India where meditation is practiced, the monks have been talking about mindfulness for thousands of years, but we are just beginning to focus on it.

In the second session, an eye fixation technique is used. Following the elicitation of a hypnotic state, some deep breathing techniques follow, and then a deepening technique involving descending a staircase. The patient is given a choice of imagining a spiral staircase or perhaps those majestic staircases like in the old mansions. Attention is drawn to differences between the techniques used in the first session and those being offered in the second. By introducing a variety of techniques, the patient will be able to have a repertoire from which to select their favorite techniques when engaged in self-hypnotic work at home. It is only logical to have an array of approaches available to meet the personality styles of an array of clients. After the induction, deep breathing, and deepening, the patient is given the following suggestions:

1. The client is told:

> The first thing we are going to do today is to review what we did in our first session. As you remember, we started off by regressing you back to your first cigarette and helping you remember all the negative bodily reactions to that very first cigarette. I suggested to you that since you only conditioned yourself to take in the negative substance for social reasons, and those social reasons no longer exist, that you could now allow your body to have its natural, instinctual reaction to cigarettes. So the suggestion was that anytime you put a cigarette to your lips or thought about smoking a cigarette, you would flash back to that very first experience … we then talked about rebelliousness and how if you needed to rebel, I suggested that you rebel against the tobacco industry, which had made their billions at the expense of our health … we talked about habit change and how the best place to break the chain is at the earliest possible link, so "don't buy cigarettes." Next we talked about those two words, the word "need" being life or death and the word "try" being a cop-out word. I suggested that you use only affirmative statements regarding your smoking cessation program, not "I'm trying to quit," but rather, "I am in the process of quitting." I also gave you three meditational statements to work on throughout the week.

2. I then use a technique which I have come to refer to as the "tobacco farm metaphor" (Stock, 1990). I tell the client:

> Today, I'll tell you a story presented by a colleague. This is a story of when he was a young medical student. He said that years ago, when he was a medical student at the University of Toronto, after being virtually locked

in by a dark and dirty winter, he was determined to get away ... to make a complete change from all that dirt and slush. He said that by March, he had assessed his options. He chose the outdoor freedom of farm life. He said that he arranged a contract for the summer on a mixed farm, which just happened to be in the middle of tobacco growing country. He added that after being stuck in the dirt and dark, it was a welcome relief. He described the broad, expansive sky, wide open spaces, and fresh air. He said there was so much he enjoyed about the life ... the arrangement between the farmer and the land. The farmer cared for the fields and they grew crops for him. He admired the arrangement with the farm animals ... in return for feeding and looking after their stalls, they would provide all kinds of amusement and work hard if called on. He talked about the beauty and strength of the work horses ... and how well they responded to control ... which was such a contrast to the noisy and smelly tractor ... and he said he still thinks about the evenings ... the work of the day completed ... and you know what it is like at 8:00 or 8:30 P.M. in June or July ... the light is golden ... slanting across the fields, casting long shadows ... the birds were quieting down ... he said he would usually take a walk from the house, down the lane to the road ... five or six dogs as companions ... it was all so peaceful and quiet. On his right, there was a 10-acre field of wheat, made more golden by the light. He said he could follow the course of the breeze across the field ... a constantly changing wave pattern ... tilting the wheat before it ... and as it did so, carrying the sound of gently rustling heads of wheat ... carrying the sweet scent of the hay ... whether it was the beauty of the time ... or the peace and quiet ... it was a golden opportunity to think about the day ... the future ... when the lane reached the road, he would usually turn right ... prolonging the walk beside the bright gold wheat ... but the character of the country-side abruptly turned somber when he reached the first of many tobacco farms in the area ... He said that if one of the dogs would dash after a groundhog ... into the tobacco field and not return ... he would have to crawl through the fence to fetch it ... walking in the furrows between the tobacco plants ... where he saw many unexpected things ... for example, the grayish stain on the leaves ... the residue of the chemicals sprayed to kill fungus ... there were regular spraying days ... and when they were downwind ... the spray made them gag ... and the farmer's 5-year-old daughter would always vomit ... Now the tobacco leaf was broad so birds flying over the field inevitably splatter the leaves with the pale yellow of their droppings ... in the slanting evening light ... the long shadows cast by the half-eaten bodies of grasshoppers ... bees ... flies ... caught and lying suspended in the cobwebs ... fastened to the leaves ... He made sure they wouldn't stick to his pants by walking around them ... And you know those little drying houses, called kilns ... sometimes if the door was left ajar and if the dog chase ended there … he found it unpleasant to enter because the frightening bats were flying wildly about … he feared they might stick in his hair … He noted that tobacco leaves hang to dry from the lines … and as they age … they wrinkle and turn yellowish brown … you can see where those bats had been sleeping … for the leaves below are streaked yellow by their feces. No matter how much he enjoyed farm life, time passed … and the day arrived when no matter how reluctant … how difficult … he had to say goodbye and get on with life. In September, he returned to medical school … strengthened by the experience … one of his first courses that semester was public hygiene … The medical students were divided into groups of ten and required to visit manufacturing facilities to check their hygienic procedures … He said that by good luck, his group was assigned to a cigarette manufacturing factory for rating … he said that they learned that by law, one out of every 200 cigarettes was removed from the line and placed under a 30-power microscope … on first looking through the eyepiece … everything is murky brown … then if you focus … you see the cut tobacco leaf … and suddenly with more precise focusing … you see other things … quite unexpected … tiny bits of pale green and pale yellow … he said he recognized these from his experiences in the summer … the tobacco leaves spattered by birds and the bat droppings on the drying tobacco leaves … and other fragments … cross-sections of insects … torsos … limbs … the insects that had been lying half-eaten in the cobwebs … he said they became quite expert in determining which was the eye of the grasshopper or fly or bee … and then the reason for the law … other pieces, dark grayish brown … these turned out to be rat droppings … they were informed that the law permitted up to six pieces per cigarette … more than six and the entire batch was destroyed … and they were curious as to how this could be … it turned out that the leaf was transported from the kilns, straight to the cutting room of the factory … no washing process … the cut leaf is then placed in bins to await wrapping … and the bins are a favorite nesting place for rodents … who leave their urine and feces … willy-nilly … He added that he now asks you to wonder just how long it takes that group of medical students to refuse to put a cigarette to their lips … let alone light up and permit penetration of that smoke and all it contains … he said that to this very day, he finds it uncomfortable to even touch a cigarette, for he knows what is inside.

Stock stressed how many of the words used in this metaphor were subtle aversive suggestions; e.g., dark and dirty, smelly, etc. These can be emphasized by changing tonal quality. Of course, some of the statements are not at all subtle, and I have found that it is not uncommon for a client to grimace when hearing them.

3.  Next the client is told:

> Now I'm going to review for you the meditational statements, but with a little more explanation *[as explained by Spiegel & Spiegel (1978)]*. As you remember, your first statement is "For my body, smoking cigarettes is a poison." Now this point is especially important because it emphasizes the fact that smoking is not so much a poison for you as it is quite specifi-cally a poison for your body. Your body is like a trusting, innocent child that has to take into it anything you put into it ... even if it is damaged by it ... like an infant, your body cannot tell you in words that it is being poisoned ... it tells you through the symptoms you experience ... the cough ... the shortness of breath ... the chest pains ... these are your body's ways of telling you it is being poisoned by cigarette smoke, so the statement is "For my body, smoking cigarettes is a poison." The second statement is "This is the only body that I have." Your body is only part of you ... most of us believe that we are more than just a physical body ... we believe that we have a mind ... and perhaps a spirit, as well as a physical body ... but the body is the precious physical plant through which you experience life on this planet ... so you're not the same as your body ... you are much more ... but you positively cannot live without it ... so the statement is "This is the only body that I have" or another way of saying it is, "I need this body to live." And the third statement is a logical deduction from one and two: "Therefore, if I want to live a long and healthy life, I must respect and protect my body by only putting into it things which are beneficial." This point emphasizes the fact that if you're going to do what you want to do in life, you need to treat your body with respect, in such a way that it can enable you to do it. For example, you can't put water in the gas tank of your car and expect it to drive you through the desert ... similarly, you can't put poison in your body without it handicapping your ability to do what you wish to do ... so the statement is "I owe my body the respect and protection of putting into it only things that are beneficial." And finally, for today ... I'm going to give you some suggestions ... and I want you to really concentrate on what I'm saying ... let your subconscious as well as conscious levels of mind activity focus on the following suggestions ... *[from Crasilneck (1990)]* ... you will no longer consciously or uncon-sciously choose to impose this undeserved burden of smoking on your heart ... your lungs ... your circulation ... and the vital organs of your body ... you will treat your body with kindness ... as if it were your closest friend ... you will find that through the immense power of your unconscious

mind, you will be able to outgrow this old, outgrown, outworn addiction ... which we now know statistically robs you of four minutes of life with every cigarette you smoke ... you will be able to give up this dirty and unhealthy habit ... as you permit yourself to rid itself of this undeserved burden of smoking ... your lungs will again become efficient ... your red blood cells will carry more oxygen to all of your vital organs ... you will feel more alert and alive and you will have a justifiable sense of pride for having worked toward and accomplished this important, healthy, worthwhile goal ... you are no longer a smoker ... you are using your own free will ... and treating yourself in a healthy and proper manner ... you will not be excessively nervous or tense ... you will not gain excessive weight ... you will exercise ... you will sleep better ... your craving for tobacco will be minimal and will decline to a zero level at a rapid pace ... all of these suggestions now firmly, deeply, permanently implanted in your sub-conscious, as well as conscious levels of mind activity ... to be used by you, as necessary ... to achieve your goal of being a non-smoker ...

# *Session 3*

As with Session 2, Session 3 begins with reviewing what we've done to date, both in the first and second sessions. I start by explaining to the patient what covert sensitization entails. It is explained that this is just the opposite of desensitization. The patient is asked to give me examples of some of the previous situations in which there was the highest probability of smoking – after a meal, with a cup of coffee, with a drink, on breaks from work, and so on. Then, the covert sensitization technique (Cautella, 1966) is employed. First of all, the patient is given one image following Cautella's approach. Ultimately, the patient imagines vomiting all over the cigarette being held, the package of cigarettes, all over their clothes, the furniture, and anything else around. Then the instruction is to imagine getting up and going to clean up, feeling so relieved being away from the cigarettes and vomit. Following that, the patient is given a technique referred to as "collapsing anchors," which is an approach presented by Zimberoff (1999). The following suggestions are given:

Now begin to get in touch with the substance that you would like to reduce or eliminate in your life ... tobacco *(this technique can be used with any substance)*. Now, I want you to open up the hand that is **not** your dominant hand ... face the palm up toward the ceiling ... and begin to bring up the urge for that substance in this hand ... now I'm going to count from 1 up to 5 ... and that urge will become stronger ... 1 ... you feel the urge for tobacco coming up now ... 2 ... it's getting stronger and stronger and stronger ... the craving for that tobacco ... 3 ... feel that urge, that craving coming up even stronger ... 4 ... it's really coming up ... and 5. How strong is that urge now from 0–10? Zero means no craving, 10 is the strongest. Raise your finger and tell me how strong it is now. Now bring your attention to your most dominant hand, the one you associate with your addictive behavior ... Turn the palm up and put into this hand, the most repulsive, gross thing you can imagine. Get in touch with whatever it is that really grosses you out. Perhaps you can see it ... notice the color and texture ... maybe it really looks gross to you ... Let's begin to bring up that most repulsive feeling ... 1 ... really increase that awful experience in your dominant hand ... 2 ... perhaps you can really smell it ... that odor is so strong! That gross disgusting smell is nearly making you sick, it is so disgusting ... 3 ... feel that slimy feeling ... using all your senses ... 4 ... the way it looks, smells, tastes, feels ... that feeling of revulsion is getting stronger and stronger ... 5 ... What number is it on now from 0–10? Zero means no feelings of disgust, 10 means the most. Tell me how strong that feeling is ... *(wait for response).* Now, in a moment, I'll count to 3 and on the count of 3, you'll clap your hands together and hold them there. This will totally collapse the original urge for tobacco ... Okay ... 1 ... 2 ... 3 ... Clap! Hold your hands together now ... just begin to feel or see this association in your mind ... the minute your hands touch, the association may begin to develop deep within your subconscious mind ... the association with that craving becomes mixed with this most repulsive image in your mind ... You can't even stand to think about that substance anymore. You immediately begin to feel sick, nauseous, uncomfortable when this substance is even talked about and you have to leave the area ... you find yourself repulsed at the thought of having to see it. Notice how that gross repulsive experience has collapsed the urge for that original substance.

At this point, I review the Spiegel techniques including the three meditational statements and the Crasilneck suggestions as presented in Session 2, after which time, the patient is brought out of the hypnotic state.

These procedures have proven to be extremely effective. When smokers ask, prior to committing to the program, about its success rates, I'll typically talk about the importance of the client's motivation. I explain that hypnosis is not a magical cure, and that for those individuals who really are not motivated to quit or are just coming because someone else suggested it, who want a magic cure, or expect me to "fix" them, the success rate is not very high. However, I continue, for those motivated individuals who really want to quit, the success rate with this program is extremely high. The patient is also told, at the expense perhaps of a negative post-hypnotic suggestion, that if, within the next year, they experience some regression and would like a "tune up," I will provide one additional session at no extra cost. Sometimes a crisis will trigger an old response, which may include going to buy a pack of cigarettes. The "booster" session might be of value at that moment. More often than not, clients do not call requesting this additional appointment. Referrals from former clients of new clients for smoking cessation suggest that there is a high success rate.

A couple of interesting successes seem noteworthy here. A local chiropractor, who happened to be a marathon runner, came to see me. He was aware that his smoking behavior and marathon running were quite inconsistent, but hadn't been able to stop smoking. I sold him the three-session package. He showed up for the second session stating that he was "cured." He said that he came to the session because it had been scheduled. We did a hypnotic session nonetheless, but he opted out of his third session (and wanted no refund). Years later, when a local newspaper was doing an article during "National Smoke-Out Week," they interviewed him. They knew he was a marathon runner (by then running ultra marathons; i.e., 50 milers) and that he used to smoke. They wanted to know how he quit. He told them, "Go interview Dr Joe Tramontana. He is the one who helped me quit." They took his advice and the article led to a great influx of new business into my practice.

Most people have heard the complaint that quitting smoking leads to an increase in irritability. A young woman called me stating that she was smoke-free after our second session. She stated, "I haven't smoked in two weeks, but I am so irritable. My husband called me a bitch, and while that is not unusual, today my best girlfriend told me I was becoming impossible to be around." I had her come in at the end of the day instead of waiting for her next scheduled appointment. We did some "uncovering work" to determine the origin of the idea that because she wasn't smoking she had to be irritable. The context came up quickly: "Well, whenever mom tried to quit she became irritable. And whenever step-dad tried to quit he became irritable." I, in turn, gave her a kind of permission to not follow suit: "You can be so pleased with your success in giving up this nasty habit and focusing on health and wellness that you will be happier than ever and not at all irritable." The next week she reported improved mood with no issues regarding irritability.

The three-session hypnotherapeutic program that was presented includes a variety of techniques and suggestions. The packaging of this program, requiring advanced payment, works on several levels, including bolstering client commitment.

Physicians sometimes prescribe pharmaceutical products, such as Zyban, which is chemically the same drug as Wellbutrin but marketed for smoking and at a higher cost, and more recently Chantrix (Varenicline), to their patients who want to quit smoking. The latter drug reportedly blocks the experience of pleasure from smoking. If patients ask, I recommend they consult their physician about a prescription. While this doesn't control for whether it is the medication or the hypnosis, or a combination thereof, the goal is abstinence. If abstinence can be achieved through a combination of approaches, I support it!

Given that smoking (and other addictions) reach into every aspect of life, it is appropriate to create interventions that support the client at various levels. Just as I work alongside AA and NA (Chapters 2 & 3), it is natural to work alongside physicians and others.

# Chapter Six

# *Focus on Weight Loss/ Obesity*

As noted in Chapter 5 on smoking cessation, offering a package of sessions has many benefits for therapists and clients. Typically, insurance companies do not pay for hypnotic weight loss programs, indicating that these are "self-help" programs. My approach of selling a "package" ensures commitment to the program and improves cash flow. First, when clients call in for services, they are offered a free consultation. Sometime I may even take out an ad in the local newspaper announcing this offer. During that 20–30 minute consultation, the client is given a questionnaire (see Appendix B). This questionnaire encompasses an extensive review of their history of weight gain, attempts to lose weight, family support, family history regarding weight, and general health issues.

Once they actually meet with the therapist, the client's weight loss goals are determined. It is explained that the loss of approximately 1½ to 2 pounds per week is considered healthy, and that the amount of weight they desire to lose will determine how many weeks the program will last. Unlike the smoking cessation program, in which each client is seen for three sessions, the weight loss program is tailored to the client's needs because unlike for smokers, where the goal is abstinence, weight loss is variable. Clients are typically seen once per week for the first three sessions, then every two weeks for the next three sessions, and then monthly until the goal weight is achieved. In other words, if a client's goal is to lose 30 lbs, at 1½ to 2 lbs per week it will likely take 15 to 18 weeks. Therefore, this client will be seen once weekly for the first three weeks, then three more times over the next six weeks, and then for two more monthly sessions, for a total of eight sessions. Someone who wants to lose 60 lbs, on the other hand, will be seen once weekly for three weeks, every two weeks over the next six weeks, and then monthly for six months, for a total of twelve sessions.

Just as in the smoking cessation program, patients are told what the hourly fee would be if they were to "pay-as-they-go." For example, at $150 per session, the fee for an eight-session program would be $1200 minus the 20% cash discount (cash/check/credit card), for a total of $960. For twelve sessions, instead of $1800 the fee would be $1440. Oftentimes, patients are also given options regarding a payment plan. For example, if they do not want the full amount charged to their credit card in one month, they might be given an option of having three consecutive monthly billings, each for one third of the total. Accepting credit card payments is very beneficial when utilizing this packaging approach.

Once again, the patients seem to be much more likely to follow through with the entire program if they pay in advance, rather than if they have to decide each week whether to come back or "do it on their own." In rare cases, if a client wants to terminate, they are given a refund, but then the discount is removed from the sessions already completed.

Another difference from the smoking cessation approach is that occasionally patients will say that they can't afford to pay a lump sum up front and would prefer to pay the full amount at each session. Because the weight loss program is a much greater total investment than the three-session smoking program, they are allowed to do so.

## *Overview*

In the consultative session, patients are given an orientation to hypnosis, as noted in Chapter 1 (i.e., "What it is and what it's not"), and then they are told that the weight loss program utilizes hypnosis for two primary functions: first, to give them posthypnotic suggestions to help them stick to a healthy eating plan, and to get them to engage in regular exercise. They are told that together we will decide on which diet is most feasible for them, and hypnotic suggestions can be geared toward helping them stay with that diet because diets can only work when people stick to them. Diet options include the Atkins' Diet, the Zone Diet, calorie counting, Weight Watchers, the South Beach Diet, and others. Clients are told:

> Most important, however, is the second facet of this approach. That is, we use hypnosis to uncover the psychological or psychodynamic reasons for your self-handicapping or self-sabotage. *Further it is explained:* Consciously, you want to be slim … consciously, you want to stick to the weight loss program … Your questionnaire indicates that you have tried many different diets on many different occasions, always with the intention of slimming. However, something must be going on at an unconscious level that causes you to self-handicap or self-sabotage your conscious motives. So the hypnosis will help us to understand why you are engaging in the self-destructive actions. And many of the patients who have reported great success through this program report that this is the basic difference between this program and others that they have attempted … that is, they now understand why they have been mis-eating in the first place.
>
> There are many different reasons that someone might gain excessive weight. One common one that many of us experience is that food, from the earliest stages of life, is associated with love and nurturance. Whether infants are breast fed or bottle fed, they are typically held close, patted, petted, and cooed to … so from the earliest days of life, food is associated with love and nurturance … if a young child falls down and scrapes his or her knee, Mama can't make the knee stop hurting, but she might give the child a cookie to take their mind off of it … so food becomes a tranquilizer … children are given treats for good behavior and success (candy, ice cream, cookies) … they're told, "Eat and you'll grow healthy, eat and you'll be strong, eat and you'll get big" … so from the earliest days of life, food is associated with all the good things in life … love, nurturance, goodness, success, health, strength, growth, tranquility … so what happens when we grow up and the world isn't treating us as well as we would like? … it's like I'll take care of me … and we start ministering to ourselves with food … of course, if you are obese, significantly overweight, or just not satisfied with your current weight, you are NOT taking care of you!

Patients are also told that there are many other reasons that people mis-eat, including sexual issues (i.e., subconscious attempts to make themselves less attractive for one reason or another), not allowing themselves to be their "best selves," self-sabotage, fear of success, and others. Festinger (1957) described some of the research on cognitive dissonance that indicated that the more energy individuals invest into a particular project, the more valuable that project becomes and their attitudes change accordingly. With weight loss, I find that by not investing fully into being their best selves, it gives them excuses for not succeeding in various life endeavors.

One of my early successes was with a young woman who was herself a mental health counselor. At the time she initiated treatment, she weighed 230 pounds. Her goal was to weigh 130 pounds. In the uncovering work, she reported that she had been a virgin until she went off to college. Once arriving at college, the first time being away from parental control, she pretty much "went wild." She had sex with anyone who asked her out. She became quite "popular" on campus, to say the least. She began to feel quite guilty and out-of-control. And then she began to eat. She gained more and more weight, and went from 130 pounds to about 180. The phone stopped ringing! She continued these eating habits through college, graduate school, and into her career. By age 30, she was up to 230 lbs. and spent most of her time, when not at work, sitting in front of the TV and eating.

Through our treatment, the patient began losing weight. When she got down to about 170 pounds, men started giving her more attention. She was concerned because of her college experiences. I instructed her, both in and out of hypnosis, that she would learn how to say "no"! "No" is a power word. The patient was told that she could and would say "no" when she meant "no" and "yes" when she meant "yes." She proudly came in shortly thereafter and described an experience. She said that a male friend had invited her on an overnight trip on his yacht. There were going to be other couples there, and she knew they would be paired off in cabins and she would be expected to sleep with him. So she just said, "No!" This story became part of the selection of case examples shared with other clients, either in or out of hypnosis.

Another recent experience is often shared with the client. In June, 2006, I was asked to serve as a judge in the Miss, Ms, and Mrs PLUS-America pageants. Contestants must be at least a size 16 to qualify for participation. The pageant director, who was a former winner, sold me on the philosophy that these women deserved the right to show that they were beautiful too. Neither swimsuit nor talent competition is a part of this contest. The participants are judged on their interviews, how photogenic they are, casual wear, and evening gown competitions. The interview is given the most emphasis, and it is stressed that it is not merely a beauty pageant. What was most noteworthy to me, however, was a subtle fact that I might not have noted on my own. A friend who did some of the contestants' hair and make-up pointed out that the three winners from the previous year's pageant, who were all present to crown the new queens, and all performed and/or participated as part of the program, were significantly smaller than their pictures from the previous year showed in the official pageant program. In other words, there were full-length pictures of all of the previous year winners, and these three women had obviously lost a considerable amount of weight. My interpretation was that because of the confidence and attention to self that came with winning the previous year, and being a national representative of the "cause," they all were inspired to focus more on physical fitness/wellness.

After this overview, patients are given a test of hypnotic suggestibility, and then they are asked if they are ready to schedule an appointment and sign up for the planned program. In some cases, they will indicate that they need to consult with their significant other regarding the cost or that they need some time to think about it. Others will schedule an appointment and pay the amount agreed upon immediately.

## *Session 1*

Various diet approaches are discussed and described, along with the pros and cons of each. After deciding on the diet plan they wish to follow, patients are shown a weight-charting technique. I draw on a blank piece of paper a rough sketch of a graph, with weight on the vertical axis and time (in days) along the horizontal axis. I roughly list their present weight at the top of the vertical axis, descending down to a manageable weight (not to absolute zero). At the level they indicated their goal weight, a horizontal line is drawn across the graph. I tell the client that this is a rough sketch for them to use as a model, but I want them to make a formal chart using graph paper or poster paper, whatever they choose. The client is told:

> I want you to weigh yourself each morning before you have had break-fast, coffee, or anything else, preferably in little if any clothing, and then plot your weight on the graph. Some weight loss programs recommend weighing only once per week, but I think you can do six days worth of damage if you only weigh weekly. I think this is especially important even when you get down to goal weight and are on a maintenance program. This charting of your progress will serve as a biofeedback process. Sure, your bathroom scale gives you feedback about your body, but seeing the progress on a chart is much more dramatic. And as you see the progress as monitored on the graph, you might give yourself a well-deserved pat on the back ... an atta-girl *(or atta-boy!)* ... and guess where I want you to keep this chart? ... On the refrigerator door! Now if you were to tell me that your highest probability of cheating is not the refrigerator, but the pantry, then I would say, then put it on the pantry door ... *Clients are told:* Some of my patients have found it helpful to also add a picture of themselves at their present weight in the upper left corner and a picture of themselves at goal weight in the lower right corner ... and if they have no pictures from the past when they were at goal weight perhaps a picture from a magazine that approximates the expected outcome ... something within reason ... not a Victoria Secret model *(most of my weight-loss clients are women; with male clients the example can be modified, perhaps to some superstar athlete)* ... but something more realistic ... and perhaps the client even attaches their own face to that body ... some who have good computer skills have used the photo programs that allow slenderizing their face to be proportionate to the body they selected.

Then hypnosis begins. As indicated in Chapter 1, I typically start with a reverse arm levitation induction, followed by deep breathing exercises, and then deepening. Once the client has taken the elevator ride or staircase or escalator to their safe, comfortable room, the following suggestions are given:

> Now I want you to imagine sitting in the safe comfortable room that we described, and on one wall of the room is a giant movie screen that covers almost the whole wall ... there are movie projectors and slide projectors. And the first thing I want you to imagine is that we are going to watch some slides ... Just a little while ago, I showed you the weight loss graph,

the chart I want you to keep. So on the first slide, I want you to imagine a giant size version of that weight chart ... Remember, on the left, the vertical axis, was weight ... the higher weight is at the top, of course ... and across the bottom is time, or days. You were instructed to plot your weight each day on the graph ... now the next slide I want you to imagine is the same slide of the graph, but now superimposed on the graph is a life-size picture of yourself at your present weight ... And see yourself in that picture with little if any clothing so you can get a good image of your physique, your body as it is now ... Nod when you have that ... Okay, now off to the lower right, where at sometime in the future you are going to achieve goal weight, I want you to see a life-size picture of yourself at your goal weight ... and nod when you have that. Okay ... it didn't take you very long. Some people have a lot of trouble imagining themselves at goal weight, but as we discussed earlier that could be because it hasn't been too long since you were there. *(This suggestion is modified when someone has been obese for many years) ...* As simple as this may seem ... what you eat and how much you exercise does, in fact, determine which of those body images you maintain ... By doing what you have been doing in terms of lack of exercise and your eating behavior, you will maintain the image in the upper left-hand corner ... By sticking to a healthy, nutritious diet that is low in fat and sugar, combined with a regular and vigorous exercise program, you will achieve and maintain the body image in the lower right-hand corner.

Now, let's turn off the slide projection and let's imagine now a movie projection. You are the star of this movie ... it is like a documentary ... It's a restaurant scene ... You are walking into a restaurant ... you're alone but feeling very independent and looking forward to a nice meal. This restaurant is different than others you've been in because this one involves being led to a table, maybe a kind of semicircular type of table where the foods are laid out in front of you already, like a feast ... a veritable feast of foods ... And the way that this restaurant works is those foods that you do not intend to eat on your diet are removed from the table so that all you are left with is a healthy, nutritious diet that you intend to eat ... and what is even more unique about this restaurant is that you don't have to say a word. It's almost as if the waiters and waitresses have ESP, because all you have to do is make a mental picture in your mind's eye of each food on that table ... as I said, a veritable feast of food ... there are high sugar and fatty foods, there are lean cuts of meat, chicken, and fish, there are salads and vegetables, low carbohydrate green and yellow vegetables ... but there are also high carbohydrate vegetables like corn and peas, potatoes ... and a lot of junk foods ... fattening things like pizza, hamburgers, some kinds of bread, and of course the desserts ... pie, cake, ice cream ... In this restaurant, you look at each food, and if it is not something good for your weight loss program, you form a picture in your mind's eye ... and put a big red X through the picture and this reminds you not to eat that food. That red X has become a universal symbol to not do something. For example, in a non-smoking area, you might see a picture of a burning cigarette with a big red X through it. Some people use the busters symbol, the circle with one line, but I like to use the red X. It means "don't do it ..." and in any language people understand that ... So for each food that you do not intend to eat, I want you to make a mental picture in your mind's eye and put a big red X through it ... And as I said, the waiters and waitresses understand and remove that from your table, one by one ... Let's start with the most obvious ones, the dessert foods ... pie, cake, ice cream, candy ... one by one they are removed from the table, all those high sugar foods ... they are high in fat too of course ... and then, perhaps the breads. And if you decide that small portions of the brown breads, like Jewish rye, pumpernickel, things like that ... small portions of that perhaps are not so bad as white bread ... And then you might get rid of the junk foods ... chips, dips, and the fast food types ... hamburgers, fried foods, fried chicken, and French fries ... The high carb veggies, one by one ... X them out. So when you're finished, all that you are going to have left is a lean diet of beef, fish, or chicken, preferably broiled, baked, or grilled ... not fried ... and only reasonable portions of those meats ... salad and salad vegetables, some low carbohydrate vegetables like the green and yellow vegetables ... spinach, broccoli, squash ... *(The foods recommended at this point may be modified to correspond more directly to whatever diet program the client and I had mutually agreed upon).* And now, see yourself sitting at that same table, with a lean meal ... but see yourself at goal weight ... Once again, what you eat does, in fact, determine which body image you maintain. By eating the feast of foods, you will maintain the higher body weight. By eating this lean meal, you will achieve and maintain goal weight ... what is even more important about this mental exercise, however, is that I want you to use this technique any time you are in a situation where you are tempted to buy or eat something not healthy for you ... you will use this mental X-ing out technique ... for example, let's say you are visiting at a friend or neighbor's house. Perhaps that person means well (sometimes they don't mean well by the way, especially if they have a weight problem ... they might attempt to sabotage your good efforts ... but we'll get into that later). Let's assume for now that this friend or neighbor means well and offers you some type of dessert food, maybe something he or she knows from the past that you have enjoyed, and you're tempted to eat that cake or pie or cookies, or whatever it might be. Perhaps you even tell yourself that you're just going to eat a tiny taste, but often times that does not work ... So if you have that urge, form a mental picture in your mind's eye and put that big red X through it ... and this is your reminder ... "No, don't do it!" And you say, "No thank you."

And finally today, I'm going to give you three meditational statements that I want you to think about each day ... then I'll teach you, when we finish, a self-hypnotic technique to practice at home. I want you to use the meditational techniques while doing your self-hypnosis, but you can also think of these statements throughout the day ... Number 1: For my mind and my body, overeating and eating fattening foods is a poison ... Now, when I first started doing this type of work, I typically said, "For my body it's a poison", because we know that being overweight causes all kinds of health problems ... increased blood pressure, high cholesterol, blood sugar problems, diabetes. It puts an extra burden on the internal organs, and also increases back pain for pain patients ... but then I came to realize that if you don't like yourself ... don't like the way you look in the mirror or the way your clothes fit or don't fit, it's also a poison for your mind. So the statement became – "For my mind and body, overeating and eating fattening foods is a poison." This is not an exaggeration. I read one report which indicated that people's life expectancy is shortened by approximately one month per pound that they are over their ideal weight plus ten. So let's say a person's ideal weight plus ten was 145 and they were 200 pounds. That would be 55 pounds over their ideal weight plus ten, which is roughly 55 months shorter life expectancy because of the extra burden that weight puts on the body ... so, the statement is, "For my body, overeating and eating fattening foods is a poison" ... Number 2: "This is the only body and mind that I have" ... a brief statement but obviously very true ... Number 3 is the logical conclusion from 1 and 2. "Therefore, if I want to live a healthy and happy life, I must respect and protect my mind and body by eating moderately and healthily." You can paraphrase these statements however you like, as long as you are getting across these three basic ideas.

Now because of time limitations I want to bring you out of the hypnotic state by counting forward from 1 to 5. At 5 that's your signal to open your eyes feeling wide awake, relaxed and refreshed, calm and confident, motivated more than ever before to achieve your weight loss goals, and confident that you are now learning the techniques that will enable you to do so. On 5, open your eyes ... 1 ... 2 ... 3 ... 4 ... and 5.

And then the person is brought out of the hypnotic state and taught a three-step self-hypnosis technique to practice at home (See Chapter 1, p. 16).

# *Session 2*

As in the earlier chapters, in the second session, I typically use an eye fixation induction and change up the deepening techniques, as well. Before the induction, the client is asked:

> Okay this is our second session ... tell me a little about how you've done since last week ... okay, so you started when? This past (day) ... and your beginning weight was_____. And your weight this morning is _____? *Congratulate weight loss. If no weight loss, stay positive:* Okay, we have work to do!

## Then the following suggestions are given:

> Alright. I want you to relax to the best of your ability ... last time, as you remember, we created tension in your arm and in the eyes ... this time, we'll localize the tension just in the eyes ... so I want you to pick out a spot on the wall or ceiling ... a spot that causes you to look up at an angle ... and very quickly you will feel tension building in your eyes ... you have already started blinking more frequently ... and each time that you blink, pay attention to the weight of your eyelids ... as they seem to get heavier and heavier ... I want you to keep staring at that spot ... feel your eyes getting really heavy ... until you're ready to let go of all of that tension ... and at that time ... close your eyes comfortably and gently ... and relax ... deeper and deeper ... and the next step is the deep breathing as we talked about last time ... breathing as you would in a really deep sleep ... slow and heavy ... slow and deep ... and now, to get you more deeply relaxed ... let's go back ... as you breathe slow and heavy like that ... once again imagine each breath as you inhale, bringing more relaxation ... and as you exhale, any remaining tensions escaping ... in with relaxation, out with tension ... relax in, tension out ... and now we're going to change the deepening techniques ... remember, last time we used the image of an elevator ride, and this time we'll change ... you'll notice that I change by design ... so that when you are practicing on your own, you can pick and choose those methods you like best ... some people prefer some techniques, while others prefer other methods ... so this time we are going to use the image of a staircase ... perhaps a spiral staircase ... or perhaps one of those majestic staircases like in the old mansions, so long as each number as I count down symbolizes for you a deeper level of hypnotic relaxation ... I want you to use all of your senses ... see yourself ... feel yourself ... sense yourself ... going deeper with each number as I count ... starting with 10 ... one being the deepest level of relaxation you

will experience for now … going down from the 10th step … down to 9 … deeper now … from 9 down to 8 … 7, and deeper … every muscle and fiber in your body relaxing further with each number … ***Continue down to 1 … then,*** as I discussed with you in the first session suggestions to stick to a healthy eating program … in today's session, we are going to work on what I call "uncovering" … that is, to uncover the subconscious motives that cause you to self-sabotage … consciously, you very much want to be slim and fit … on a conscious level you want to stick to your diet … and you want to lose weight and be physically healthy … but something is going on at a subconscious level that causes you to self-handicap … to self-sabotage … to behave in a manner inconsistent with your conscious goals … so I want you to imagine once again being in the safe, comfortable room that we described last time … remember that on one wall was a giant movie screen … the last time, we looked at the slide image of your weight chart and your before-and-after images … we also looked a the movie of the restaurant scene … and the part about X-ing out foods not in your eating plan, your weight loss program … today, however, we are going to look at another film … and this film is about your life … everything that you have ever experienced is stored on this film … actually, the film is a symbolic representation of your own subconscious mind … you see, your subconscious mind knows everything about you … everything you have ever seen, heard, felt, sensed … it is all stored there … your subconscious is like a memory bank … like a computer … in fact, we sometimes refer to the subconscious as being like a "biological computer" … everything you have ever experienced is stored there … and all we need do is access that computer … and the way we access it is through hypnosis … so in just a moment, I'm going to count backwards from 5 to 1, and as I count, I want you to imagine the film rewinding … and when I get to 1, I want you to be at some very significant experience in your past … some experience related to the problems that you are having as an adult with weight … now, I don't want you to think about it … analyze it … assess it … monitor it … rather, just let the information flow … we call this technique "developing an affect-bridge" … It means that if there is something going on at present, and we can find an earlier beginning or origin of that problem, that bridges the gap, so to speak … that affected this … and the reason we use a movie screen … a technique we call hypnoprojection … is that if there was something very negative … traumatic … scary … whatever … you don't have to relive it … you can see it as if watching a film … in fact, this is like a documentary … a documentary about your life … but you're also the narrator of this documentary … so you don't have to relive it … you can see it as if on screen … in just a moment, I'm going to start counting … as I count, imagine the film rewinding … when I get to 1, I want you to imagine a scene coming into focus on that screen … and

> then I'll ask you to talk to me and tell me what you see, hear, feel, sense, or know … on 1 … let the picture come into focus … now lets rewind the film … going back in time … 5 … rewinding … 4 … seeking … scanning … 3 … 2 … and 1 … all the way back to 1 … now imagine a picture coming into focus … and when you have something in your mind, let me know by nodding your head gently … what comes to you? … *If the patient comes up with something, good! If not, go on:* Sometimes when people do this for the first time, they see a blank screen … or maybe they see just blackness … or maybe they see a lot of different colors all jumbled up that don't make any sense … imagine we can adjust the fine focus … and have some picture come into focus on that screen … concentrate … let your creative mind work for you … imagine a picture coming into focus … and that picture is going to tell us some significant event in your past related to problems in your adult life … at the present time … with weight … and what comes to you?

Pause while patient describes the picture. If the patient sees something, which often happens, we will then investigate that. But if not, then there are other avenues we can take, such as focusing on the first time they ever realized that they were overweight. For example, I might investigate whether the patient was teased by someone about their weight (relatives, peers, et al), or I might ask when was the first time the patient felt "different" from peers. An approach I learned in a codependency workshop many years ago, which was referred to by the presenter as being a technique from the literature on healing the wounded child within (Whitfield, 1987), might also be appropriate:

> When you are upset at the present time, where do you physically feel that emotional upset? For some people, they might describe heaviness in their chest, or difficulty breathing, or head pounding, or pain in their stomach … when you are most upset in the present time, where do you physically feel the emotional upset? *After the patient describes where they physically feel the upset* … Okay … now I'm going to count backward from 5 to 1, and when I get to 1, I want you to go back to the very first time that you felt those feelings in your stomach (or head, or chest, etc.)

It is rare that a client does not come up with any memories that relate to the weight issues. However, in those rare cases, we can actually use the lack of developing an affect-bridge by stating:

Good. So apparently there are no psychological reasons for you to hold on to this extra weight. Do you agree? ... Since there are no psychological reasons for you to maintain the weight, it is apparent that you are now ready to go on with the rest of the weight loss program.

An adjustment might also need to be made for a person who only recently gained weight:

Many different factors go into excessive weight gain ... a person who put on the weight recently is different than one who always had the problem, or has been up and down for many years ... gains and loses ... but the fact is, and to your benefit, experts typically say that new weight (even a couple of years would be considered new in terms of a lifetime) ... is easier to lose than weight that you carried for many years ... so that's the good news ...

## *Session 3*

In Session 3, hypnosis is often elicited using an eye roll technique (once again, to reinforce the idea that there are many different techniques used to usher one into the hypnotic state). The deep breathing and deepening techniques follow. After using the elevator and staircase images in the first two sessions, Session 3 incorporates an escalator or descending a gently sloping hill down to the ocean or to a valley. In Session 3, we do a brief review of Sessions 1 and 2 and what we learned in those sessions, followed by the client being given the metaphor entitled "tending the garden," and then relaxing scenes, including a beach scene, a woods scene, with the metaphor of a logjam.

I received the following "tending the garden" metaphor as a handout at a workshop many years ago. Over the years, clerical assistants have typed and re-typed it, and at some point, the piece was separated from the author's name and a reference. I have searched extensively, but as of this time the author of that handout is unknown to me. However, I have used it for many years and believe it is an excellent metaphor to assist clients in making healthy eating choices. The client is told:

As you relax and concentrate, let your imagination open and allow yourself to picture a large open field surrounded by trees ... it is a beautiful spring day ... the sun is shining ... the sky is blue ... and you feel a warm, gentle breeze, and the sound of song birds comes to you clearly ... the earth beneath your feet is soft and moist ... new grass is just coming up ... a beautiful yellow-green ... you begin to wander ... not wonder ... wander ... or maybe both, wander and wonder ... across the field ... and as you do, you see ... just at the edge of the field nearest you ... a wooden shed ... you wonder idly what it contains ... you continue walking down the center of the field toward the far side ... where you can perceive some- thing shining in the sun ... like water ... but your attention is distracted by the grass, flowers, and weeds ... the arrangement of the weeds seems to hint at cultivation ... they seem to be arranged in square beds ... all the way down both sides of the center, grassy section of which you are walk- ing ... you turn around and investigate ... there are beds all around you ... so then you turn aside to investigate the nearest of these beds ... on your right ... you kneel down and try to examine the weeds and amongst them you discover the unmistakable early shoots of tomato plants, but they are so choked with weeds that they will really never have a chance to grow ... you rise and move to the next bed and you discover the tiny fern-like prongs of carrots, also half smothered by weeds ... you become excited and expectant ... and you cross to the beds on the other side of the field ... examining each one ... crossing back to check all the beds in the field until you arrive back at the place you started ... and in each bed, you find a different vegetable or fruit struggling to grow through the enveloping weeds ... Now, alerted, you examine more closely the trees around the field and you discover they are fruit trees ... apple, pear, plum, peach, cherry ... and just on the edge of the orchard are vines struggling to produce grapes ... the trees need pruning in order to produce and all the vines desperately require weeding, feeding, and cultivating ... what a waste to let the weeds take over ... you feel a certain sense of respon- sibility toward this field ... which is not surprising ... it is your field, after all ... planted years ago and then abandoned ... and now you remember what the shed contained ... tools and fertilizer ... you begin to feel an urgency to return the field to its proper condition ... remove the weeds ... cultivate the beds ... to water and tend the young plants and bring them back to health ... and productivity ... you hurry to the shed, rummaging in your pocket for the key to the padlock ... the key you have carried with you for all these years ... but had forgotten ... you insert the key in the lock and turn ... it is stiff, but a little graphite and regular use would ease the stiffness. You enter the shed, knowing exactly where to find all the tools you require ... the hoe ... the small hand spade and cultivator ... watering cans ... a basket for the refuse you are going to pull out of the beds ... and your old gardening gloves ... a little dusty, but soft and comfortable and familiar ... you brush off the dust ... you put them on, and they feel very good as if they are part of you ... you gather your tools ... load them into the wheelbarrow and wheel them off to the first bed ... as you kneel ... pulling handfuls of weeds away from the struggling tomato plants you feel good ... comfortable ... as though you have come home ... you breathe deeply the rich aroma of the soil and the plants ... the smell of Spring is full of promise ... you proceed quickly and in a very short time, you have cleared most of the weeds from that bed ... as you add the fertilizer to the soil ... you find yourself imagining the plants as they will be ... loaded with red, ripe, luscious tomatoes ... full and juicy ... your mouth waters at the thought ... you can't wait to sink your teeth into one ... you can almost taste it now ... but one more chore remains before you can proceed to the next bed ... you must water the tomatoes ... you remember now what the sparkling area is at the other end of the field ... it is a small lake ... clean and clear ... fed by the snow melt and a mountain stream ... and you pick up the watering can and walk toward it ... you kneel at the bank ... and see your reflection just as you saw in the mirror this morning ... but something looks different ... your face seems just a little less full ... your clothes just a little looser ... you like the change and you smile ... and suddenly there is a ripple ... and when the ripple disappears you see another, different reflection ... it is still recognizably you, but so different from the first ... you see yourself slim and thin ... and graceful, just as you've always wanted to be *... (or "just as you once were")* ... and you gaze at the picture of yourself ... engraving it indelibly in your memory ... then, just as suddenly as it appears ... it is gone ... you get the water from the lake to fill the watering can and as you carry it back to the tomatoes ... you're thinking about that wonderful picture ... and you realize that each time you successfully reclaim another bed, another orchard, from the weeds and the neglect ... your reflection will more closely resemble that ideal ... until one day, all the beds and all the vines and all the trees will be loaded with fruit and you will be what you wish yourself to be ... as you saw yourself in that moment at the lake ... each time you do your self-hypnotic work at home, you reclaim another part of your garden ... each time you will see the results ... as your image more and more closely approximates your goal ... and each time you find yourself impatient for the produce of your garden ... the promise of each bed and tree making your mouth water for the fruit ... from the beds which you are tending ... and when you emerge, you will retain the desire for that produce and it will be reflected in the foods you prefer.

## *Relaxing Scenes*

I want you to continue to relax ... further ... deeper ... let's concentrate on an even deeper relaxation by doing some visual imagery ... I want you to imagine some scenes as I describe them to you ... some relaxing scenes ... now when you practice at home, you can pick and choose scenes that you like or that you've actually experienced that are peaceful and calming ... but for now I want you to focus on some scenes that I'll give you. *[This imagery is presented in Chapter 2, pp. 25–27 but repeated here for those readers interested in weight loss approaches who might not have read the chapter on alcohol abuse.]*

First, a beach scene, perhaps a beautiful, spring or summer day, just sitting on a beach towel or blanket, or in a recliner of some sort ... appreciate the beautiful scenery ... the beautiful weather ... you feel the warm sunlight on your skin, but there is a nice breeze coming off the water ... and there are some sailboats out in the water ... it's a very calm day ... and you notice how effortlessly they glide through the water, pushed by the gentle breeze ... perhaps there are some seagulls flying near the water's edge, and you notice how they too, seem to move so effortlessly on the wind currents ... perhaps a ship on the horizon ... now we know that it takes a lot of power to motor a ship, but it's the efficient use of power that causes it to appear effortless ... perhaps a jet plane in the sky ... it too takes a tremendous amount of power, but again, it is the efficient use of power that causes this apparent effortlessness ... These are your key words ... **efficiency** and **effortlessness**.

Okay, let's go to a second scene ... this one is a woods scene ... perhaps a beautiful fall morning ... one of those fall mornings when you feel that certain crispness in the air ... you're walking in the woods ... perhaps a state park type setting ... enjoying the beautiful sights ... maybe the leaves are turning colors ... the birds are chirping ... enjoying the beautiful sights and sounds and smells of the forest ... so peaceful and calm ... as you walk down the path, you notice an area up ahead where there are no more trees ... as you get closer, you see the reason is that there is a body of water running through it ... like a narrow river or wide stream ... as you get closer you see how crystal clear and clean and flowing is that body of water ... so clean and clear you can see your reflection ... almost like a mirror image ... and you notice how reliably and predictably the water flows ... efficiently and effortlessly ... there are those key words again ... **efficiency** and **effortlessness** ... you may notice near the water's edge, where the water is only an inch or two deep, some rocks or pebbles ... you notice how the water just goes around them and over them ...

perhaps some boulders out in the middle, and there, too, the water goes around them, continuing on its path ... you decide to continue walking down that riverbank ... and you come to a bridge ... a walking bridge ... the kind you might see in a state park ... a wooden bridge with a curved handrail ... sometimes they are called "foot bridges" ... you decide you want to cross over to the other side ... you step up onto the bridge ... but as you get halfway across, you notice that something has gone awry ... the water below is not clean and clear and flowing anymore ... it is becoming muddied and dirty and is backing up ... you investigate and see what has happened ... apparently some logs were floating down this body of water and became lodged under the bridge causing a logjam ... as you investigate even more closely, you see that there is one log that is bigger than the rest ... it's the main problem ... it became wedged under the bridge causing the other logs to back up behind it ... I want you to really concentrate on that big log ... and see if you see anything written on that log ... it might be written, or engraved, or inscribed ... it could be a word ... maybe even a name ... it could be a phrase, or a whole sentence or more ... concentrate on this log ... see if there is anything written ... and whether you see something or not ... some people do and some don't ... what's most important is the next step ... and that is ... you make a conscious decision to take matters into your own hands to remedy this problem ... you cross over to the other side and you find a board, pipe, or tree limb ... something you can use as a lever ... and you set about the process of freeing up this logjam, whether it involves leaning down from the bridge, leaning out from the bank, or even wading into the water, you set about the process of freeing up the logjam ... you use the board or pipe or lever ... and you pry loose that big log ... and to your surprise, it loosens rather easily ... and once it loosens, it begins floating again, under the bridge ... and the other logs follow suit ... you walk back onto the bridge, and you watch as the logs float off into the distance ... and the farther away they get, the smaller they seem, and the smaller they seem, the farther away they are, until they get so very far away, they look like little tiny specks in the distance ... finally, they round a bend, and you don't see them at all anymore ... you know they still exist, somewhere, but no longer in your field of experience ... and you look back into the water, and once again it is clean, and clear, and flowing ... You see your reflection in the water ... You might even see yourself smiling, being proud of having taken remedial action to fix this problem ... and perhaps you see yourself slim, just as you want to be.

Now as you may or may not have figured out, this is a metaphor, full of symbolism. The body of water symbolizes one's path through life. And we started at first when it was clean and clear and flowing ... The little rocks and pebbles represent minor setbacks, minor frustrations, but life's force, life's energy just continued around and over them, continuing on its way ... Now the boulders represent bigger problems, but even there, life's energy kept flowing, undaunted ... now the logjam represents a major blockage, and the big log, of course, would be the biggest problem ... By the way, did you see anything written on that big log *(Whether the client saw something or not, their response can be interpreted to the advantage of the process)* ... As I said earlier, the most important thing is the next point ... that is, your decision to take remedial action to resolve this problem. That could be symbolic of coming here. Perhaps I am the lever, or maybe hypnosis is the lever, but in any event, you made the decision and took action to remedy the problem, and as the logs floated off into the distance, this was symbolic of alleviation of the problems.

At this point, the patient is brought out of the hypnotic state. They are told that the next appointment, according to the schedule, would be in two weeks, since this was the third of the three once-weekly sessions. If, for some reason, the client prefers not to skip a week, the change can be accommodated.

After Sessions 1 through 3, the patient is instructed to practice these techniques at home. On occasions where the client reports having difficulty doing self-hypnosis, a recording is made. I prefer to make this recording while the client is actually in session, so that the hypnotic suggestions are specific to them (rather than the generic recordings that can be bought in a bookstore).

## *Session 4*

In Session 4, the client is told to use any of the previous induction techniques, whether it involves staring at the hand, staring at a spot on the wall, or an eye roll technique, to enter into a hypnotic state. After a brief review of what was covered in the first three sessions, some work is done regarding what I refer to as "overcoming the fear of getting slim." Many people have psychological reasons for resisting weight loss, one of which might be because there is some secondary gain for not being one's "best self." Perhaps the client is looking for an excuse to explain why they didn't pursue that outside sales job. Perhaps the client creates the "reason" they are unable to attract the particular partner that they ultimately desire. The variations are many. An example is sometimes shared with the client.

> I had a patient a few years ago who was a beautiful young woman. In fact, I thought that her face looked a lot like Catherine Zeta-Jones. She reported that she felt she was about 30 pounds overweight. She also reported that relationships never worked out for her. It turned out that the typical relationship of this single female was with married men. There was always the promise that the man would leave his wife for her, but it never happened. Under hypnosis, what came out was that the 30 pounds of extra weight was her rationale for why these men never left home for her: "If I were at goal weight, then they would have chosen me, but I'm overweight." This rationale was less threatening to her than to say, I'm as physically perfect as I can be, and he still didn't leave her for me.

Of course, cognitive behavioral therapy ensued for this patient regarding her "choices" in partners.

## Overcoming the Fear of Getting Slim

> In the past, we have done some work with hypnotic regression; that is, going back into your past to look at possible early origins of your weight concerns. Today, however, we are going to project into the future ... so I want you to see yourself, at some time in the not-too-distant future, when you have achieved goal weight ... and I want you to see yourself at some social function where there are others who will notice and comment on your new level of fitness ... see yourself wearing something that really shows off your new, slimmer figure. For example, it might be a cocktail party at which you are wearing a dress that really shows your figure ... or perhaps a pool party or a beach party ... *(These images are adjusted accordingly for men, with a focus on physique)* ... imagine yourself slim, trim, physically fit, just the way you've always wanted to be, at goal weight ... people notice, and they compliment you ... now, tell me where you see yourself and what is going on ...

After the patient describes the situation, the party, the function, whatever, they are told:

> Well that sounds great, everything is just like you would like it to be, isn't it? You look good, you feel happy ... you have more energy, you are alive, and others are complimenting you, isn't this great? ... NOW, I want you to

really concentrate on this scene! I want you to find something **bad** about the scene.

Sometimes, people have trouble finding something bad. Oftentimes, however, they quite easily come up with interesting material. There are some women who say that they are in business and want to be accepted for their brains and not their looks, or that their spouse is jealous, or that girlfriends now become jealous, and so these issues are dealt with. Within a short time, I had two such clients. One was in her early forties and weighed 170 pounds, but wanted to weigh 140 again. The other was in her early thirties and weighed 150 pounds. She wanted to weigh 120 again. Both were in business with their husbands, and both reported that their husbands were "jealous" anytime they received attention from other men.

Regarding the spouse being jealous, it is often the case that the spouse is already insecure about possibly losing his wife to another before any weight loss occurred. This insecurity will sometimes lead to the spouse's attempts (conscious or unconscious) to sabotage the client's weight loss efforts (e.g., bringing home desserts or candy). So if the client is 30 pounds overweight, and her husband is already insecure, I might say:

> Well, apparently being 30 pounds overweight hasn't worked in preventing him from being insecure, so if that is your goal, perhaps you should gain another 30 pounds, so he can be certain that other men are not flirting with you.

The client will resist this suggestion and be reinforced for that assertive resistance. I will then respond:

> Of course, that is ludicrous! And since that is ludicrous, it makes no sense to hold onto the present 30 pounds overweight either!

## Session 5

In Session 5, the patient is introduced to the technique described in Chapter 3 on Drug Abuse, which I refer to as "Space Travel Meditation." The only difference is that the information to be gleaned from this educational trip into outer space is to get advice from this all-wise being (or *inner adviser*) regarding the causes of the maladaptive eating patterns, resistance to losing weight, and any other insights into the problem. Following this "uncovering" technique, of course, is to get counsel/advice from this wise being regarding the steps that need to be taken to remedy the problem. Often, the wise being's advice covers aspects we have already discussed, but the additional counsel puts an exclamation point to the perspective. Sometimes the client will describe having met Jesus, or some supernatural being, sometimes a deceased relative, such as a grandparent, whose advice they respected. Whatever the client comes up with is followed by a brief discussion of the idea that we all have much more wisdom, often in our unconscious or subconscious mind, than we realize. The example given is that of going somewhere to learn something and leaving thinking, "I knew that!" *The answer is that we often know much more than we realize that we know. So the Space Travel Meditation is a technique to channel information from our own unconscious mind, through the all-wise being, back to our conscious mind.*

## Session 6

Just as at the beginning of all the sessions, the patient is asked how they are doing, including their current weight, new insights, pitfalls, and so forth. In Session 6, after reviewing some of the previous sessions, I introduce the patient to an adaptation of the metaphor of the World Class Visualizer presented by Poulos and Smith (1998) in their sports medicine CEU Conference. In this case, the story is adapted to what this world class expert would say regarding the patient's weight loss attempts and how they might be different from the way the patient may be looking at it through their own eyes and with their own brain. The client is told:

> I want you to imagine that you have a secret garden ... and I want you to imagine entering that garden, and then I want you to describe to me everything you see.

Give the client a few minutes, and they will typically describe flowers, trees, perhaps colors and textures, paths through the garden, perhaps a pond. Then I say:

> Very good! Now I want you to imagine that you could put on the head of a world class visualizer ... perhaps a famous artist ... or an inventor ... Einstein was said to be a world class visualizer ... and imagine that you can now see that garden through this world class visualizer's eyes and with the benefit of his or her brain ... and describe the garden to me again using the world class visualizer's eyes and brain.

Typically the client describes the garden in much greater detail. For example, they might see not just the flowers, but bees pollinating the flowers, not just the trees, but the texture of the bark, not just the pond, but goldfish swimming in the pond, and so forth. Then, the client is told:

> You have been seeing your weight loss efforts for so long through your own eyes and with your own brain ... I now want you to imagine seeing it through the eyes of and with the brain of a world class nutrition and fitness expert ... someone who knows exactly how to counsel you regarding what will work for you in terms of an eating plan and exercise plan. And I want now for you to adopt this viewpoint as your own ... for, after all, it really did come from your creative mind.

## *Session 7*

In this session, after reviewing progress and some of the materials from earlier sessions, the client might be introduced to a technique from neuro-linguistic programming (Bandler & Grinder, 1976) involving visualization regarding their weight using a fading-in, fading-out approach. For example, they are told:

> Imagine sitting in that comfortable room that we described in our first hypnotic session ... and looking at a wide-screen TV with a picture-in-picture feature. I want you to see yourself at your beginning weight on the main screen, but in a tiny insert in the lower right-hand corner see yourself at goal weight. Then we are going to fade out the old and fade in the new ... the big picture, how you used to be will become smaller and smaller, dimmer and dimmer ... the insert, how you want to be becomes bigger

and bigger, brighter and brighter ... since you have already been making progress toward your goal, at some point the big picture will be an exact replication of how you see yourself when you look in the mirror now ... but the fading continues, so that you eventually see the big picture, how you want to be, covering almost the whole screen ... and all that is left of the old image is a tiny, dim insert in the upper left-hand corner ... rather than get rid of it completely, we will keep it up there, like on a shelf, just to remind you of what can happen if you are not cautious about maintaining the new image.

The patient may also be given scenes that involve eating, in which the split-screen approach is used – seeing themselves first of all on the major part of the screen, the way they used to approach food, and then in the tiny insert in one corner seeing the way they would like to do it. The fading-in, fading-out approach would then be employed.

The number of sessions for which the client has contracted determines where to go from here.

## *Session 8*

Session 8 might be devoted entirely to a review of previous sessions, in order to anchor the understandings and techniques. However, if there are additional sessions to follow because the client has contracted for more sessions and/or has not reached goal weight, the additional sessions will often incorporate the techniques from prior sessions. If the client only contracted for eight sessions, but has not reached their goal, investigation might ensue regarding an action plan. This plan might involve suggestions for their self-hypnotic work. In some cases, the client might opt to continue in treatment. When this is the case, I typically give them the option of paying on a per session basis or contracting for another, usually smaller package of sessions using the discounting method described earlier in this chapter.

Since attending Ewin's workshop (2008), I have also successfully employed his ideomotor questioning technique with two weight-loss clients. In both cases, the clients were able to provide information that helped uncover additional psychodynamics of the maladaptive eating habits. In each case, the client gave more information than they had in Session 2, during which I had used my standard uncovering techniques.

Further sessions often incorporate storytelling either in or out of hypnosis. One story is about the time I participated in a panel discussion regarding weight loss programs.

> I, along with a nutritionist, and representatives from Weight Watchers, Overeaters Anonymous (OA), TOPS (Take Off Pounds Sensibly), and Nutri-systems participated in the program, which was promoted by a local hospital. I talked about hypnotically enhanced weight loss, of course. I told of an experiment I had read a long time ago about a group who worked on a task during which they were told they couldn't wear watches (for a disguised reason), and there were no windows in the room. There were clocks on the wall. The group was made up of two distinct subgroups. One group was fit and trim, the other group was considerably overweight. The morning session ended at noon, at which time they all went to lunch. While out of the room, the clocks were exchanged for clocks rigged to run fast. So after they returned to the task, when the clock said 6:00 p.m., it was really only 4:00 p.m. Almost every member of the overweight group, complained: "I'm hungry. It's time to eat." Members of the slim group responded quite differently: "Well I know it is 6 o'clock, but for some reason I'm just not hungry." The interpretation was that people who tend to maintain slimness are controlled by internal bodily needs, whereas people who tend toward obesity are controlled by external stimuli. The external stimuli could be time of day, the availability of food, etc.
>
> At that point, the speaker from Weight Watchers spoke up. She said: "I can definitely relate to that. I have been at goal weight now for about eight years. But just recently I was having lunch with my husband. He has never had a weight problem. I ate a salad, while he ate a burger and fries. He left three French fries on his plate. I asked: 'Aren't you going to finish your French fries?' To which he responded: 'I'm full.' My next question was: 'How can you leave just three French fries?' He answered: 'And that is why you have always had a problem and I haven't!'"

I typically do not use the aversion techniques (covert sensitization or collapsing anchors) with weight loss patients. These techniques can be effective with smokers, alcoholics who opt for the abstinence model, drug addicts, pathological gamblers or any addiction for which the goal is abstinence. With eating, however, the goal is to develop healthier eating habits. On the other hand, if there are specific foods that are described as problematic, aversion techniques might be employed. For example, one woman said that her only problem in sticking to her program was chocolate. I gave her the following suggestions:

> I want you to remember a time in your past when you ate too many sweets, maybe as a child, at a circus ... you had cotton candy, ice cream, Crackerjacks, and chocolate ... and you became very sick to your stomach and had to vomit ... can you remember such an experience (*client acknowledges and describes the situation*) ... from now on ... and until you reach goal weight and maintenance, anytime you see or even think about eating chocolate, you will flash back to that experience at the____, and become just as violently ill as you were then.

The client returned the next week and reported the following experience. "I was in the supermarket shopping and I accidentally went down the candy aisle. When I saw chocolates, I gagged and felt like I was going to puke right on the spot. I did a u-turn with my buggy and the bad feelings went away."

Many clients have reported significant success in achieving their weight loss goals and maintaining these goals, and most relate their success to "understanding why they were mis-eating." My experience has been that those clients who are most successful in losing the weight and keeping it off are the ones who have also incorporated regular exercise into their programs. I highly reinforce exercise. One reason, perhaps, is that exercise is an "active" behavior, whereas not eating certain foods is more passive or, at least, less "proactive." This sense of passivity can be offset by telling patients that putting a lot of time and energy into eating healthy is a way to make their dieting program proactive rather than passive. Further, the literature on the use of exercise as treatment for depression corroborates the idea that exercise can play a big part in clients achieving a higher level of self-esteem.

Sometimes, clients will make all kinds of excuses for not exercising. One that comes to mind was offered by a woman who was a business executive. She had an important job, often worked late, and had a 45-minute commute to and from work. She said that she had a treadmill in her home and used to walk on it while watching the news, but just never seemed to have time anymore. It just so happened that I had a recent copy of *Runner's World Magazine* in my waiting room that had a picture on the cover of President George Bush running, with his Secret Service Agents. The cover story related how he ran three miles every morning and actually got some work done while running by having aides run with him. I asked the client: *Are you busier than the President of the United States?* To which she responded: *Alright, damn it, I'll do it!* The weight started coming off.

In summary, this chapter describes a business plan of packaging the sessions and requiring advanced payment or at least advanced partial payment for the entire program. The number of sessions in the program is determined by the amount of weight the client wishes to lose. Scripts and techniques for the first eight sessions are given. For very obese clients who need more than eight sessions, some of the earlier scripts are repeated in subsequent sessions. Suggestions regarding exercise are also incorporated.

Patients have often reported that finally understanding *why* they mis-eat has been crucial in their weight loss. Many of these clients had reported in the pre-treatment questionnaire that there had been many previous attempts and programs geared toward weight loss, but with little success or little sustained benefits. The combination of post-hypnotic suggestions to reinforce a healthy eating and exercise program, along with this psychological understanding of their old, maladaptive patterns appears much more effective in maintaining the clients' goals.

# Chapter Seven

# The Panorama

I began in Chapter 1 by describing the "Lens" through which I see hypnosis/hypnotherapy in working with addictions. But there is a much broader picture that needs to be addressed using these economically efficient and effective techniques.

Addictions appear to be a very ripe field for hypnosis and hypnotherapy. Most addicts are looking for the "quick fix," of course, and while we cannot provide magical cures, hypnotic techniques are certainly very effective in dealing with addictions.

There are many addictions not covered in this book, including sexual addictions, shopping, stalking, pornography, the internet, etc. Sixteen million Americans are said to suffer from compulsive sexual behavior. Internet addiction, perhaps an impulse-control disorder, like gambling, is on the rise. And it is estimated that 1 in 20 Americans is a compulsive shopper. The statistics across the board are startling.

One of the things that I learned from a colleague many years ago is that in Step One of the 12-Step programs, anything can be substituted for alcohol. A person can say: "I came to realize that I was powerless over alcohol, or drugs, gambling, sex, food, tobacco, Mary, Sam, etc ... and that this substance, activity, or person makes my life unmanageable.

When we add to the addiction puzzle the complications created by cross-addictions, the picture often becomes more treatment resistant. Just recently I saw a young man seeking help for a sexual addiction. He would snort cocaine and then make obscene phone calls. When a 16-year-old niece "busted" him, he came in for treatment. It did appear that the sexual addiction was primary, but cocaine was added to the mix as a stimulus to engage in the behavior.

Sometimes, too, an addiction is the primary problem but is hidden behind some other presenting problem. For example, in one of my EAP contracts a number of years ago, at a regional IRS site, it was noted that the number of clients seeking services for addictions was much lower than population statistics would have led us to expect. In a quarterly roundtable discussion between myself, our counselor for that area, and IRS administrators, this issue was discussed. Although many employees called requesting services for marital problems, family problems, or financial problems, few called about alcohol, drugs, or gambling. One of the IRS staff members, who happened to be the Center's budget and financial counselor, spoke up. Her job was to counsel IRS employees who were having financial problems, and she said: "Anytime I talk with an employee who is making a decent income and whose spouse is making a decent income, but they say they just can't seem to make ends meet, I slam my hand down on the desk and say, 'All right, who is addicted to what?' Somebody is spending too much money on something: alcohol, drugs, gambling, shopping, fishing (boats and gear are expensive), hunting, something!" She was on target because addictions are sneaky and sometimes the therapist might not be immediately aware, at intake, that addictions are at the center of the presenting issue.

In addition, many of the individuals with gambling, drug and other addictions turn out to be adept "con-men" or "con-women." Whether they learned to con to cover up their addictions (denial), to avoid scrutiny, escape punishment, or whether they are sociopaths independent of their addictions may not be immediately clear. And, of course, the con games accomplish multiple goals. All of this is to say that the nature and manifestation of addiction is complex and multifaceted. Fortunately, hypnosis is an approach – used alone or in tandem with other paradigms – that is flexible, permissive, and non-threatening, thus giving the therapist the power to address a wide range of variables and offer relief.

The packaging techniques described in the chapters on smoking and weight loss can greatly improve the chances of clients following through on their commitments, not to mention enhancing the cash flow of your practice. Once patients are engaged in the treatment, a positive cycle of commitment – success – renewed commitment often ensues.

Many hypnotherapists rely heavily on using previously published scripts for particular disorders. After all, we often tend to think, "Why reinvent the wheel?" Oftentimes, as we become more experienced, we modify or adapt others' scripts to work with our particular style. Although I have stressed the importance of developing more techniques for hypnotically enhanced addictions treatment, one might also incorporate some of the more generic scripts already described by other practitioners. For example, Wright's (1987) strategies for overcoming pleasure-producing habits might be modified for any of the addictions in the five chapters in this volume, as well as the other addictions mentioned above which were not addressed. In fact, I have used his "strategy of positive future consequences" in my work. This approach highlights the long-term rewards to be realized from overcoming the habit. For example, with smokers, there is a strong focus on the benefits of breathing better rather than on the pain of labored breathing, a focus on the lightness and increased energy resultant from weight loss versus a focus on the ills of obesity, and so on. This is the flipside of confronting patients with long-term negative consequences, which has been demonstrated here in all of the chapters. Hypnotic practitioners can no doubt use their creative minds to find many ingenious ways to develop scripts for some of the lesser-studied addictions.

The power of the human mind never ceases to amaze me; something that has been shown again and again in the various successes in meeting the challenges of the above addictions. Early on in my work with smoking cessation, there was one case that really demonstrated the power of the human mind. A recovering alcoholic, who was very active in AA, attending many meetings per week, never attended the "non-smoking meetings." After my standard three-session package, she reported that she had cut down from almost three packs per day to only four cigarettes daily. I attempted to reinforce the idea that this was tremendous progress, but she was unhappy that she had not quit totally (because of her strong AA bent, abstinence was the only acceptable outcome for her). I saw her for an additional session. She had proven to be a very highly hypnotizable individual. I gave her the following suggestion:

> From now on anytime you put a cigarette to your lips, you will feel a hot, burning sensation on your lip.

She called me a few days later. Despite the fact that she was still spending a lot of time in smoky AA meetings, she stated that not only had this last suggestion worked in helping her to quit smoking totally, but she had actually developed a blister on her lip where she felt the cigarette was hot and burning.

In my very first ASCH training session in 1978, one of the presenters stated: "Hypnosis will not only change your practice, it will change your life." Some 30 years later, I have found – and continue to find – that the possibilities are limitless!

# Appendix A

# *Example of Smoking Cessation Inventory*

Name:_____ Age: _____ Date: _____

Marital Status:_____ Occupation: _____

Is your work stressful?
- ❏  No
- ❏  Moderately
- ❏  Very

How many cigarettes do you smoke in a day? _____

At what age did you start smoking? _____

What do you get from smoking?
- ❏  It relaxes me
- ❏  It gives me a confidence boost
- ❏  It's a prop
- ❏  It helps me to concentrate
- ❏  It's an excuse for a break
- ❏  It helps me avoid being angry or upset
- ❏  Other:

When do you smoke?
- ❏  On awakening
- ❏  With tea/coffee
- ❏  Driving
- ❏  At work
- ❏  At breakfast
- ❏  After meals
- ❏  On the phone
- ❏  In the bed
- ❏  Other:

What do you like about smoking? _____

_____

Do others in your life smoke? If so, who? _____

When?
- ❏ At home
- ❏ Socially
- ❏ At work
- ❏ Other:

Do you know someone who has died from a smoking related disease?
- ❏ Yes
- ❏ No

Has your doctor mentioned your smoking?
- ❏ Yes
- ❏ No

Have you had any worrying symptoms?
- ❏ Yes
- ❏ No

Do you have any health problems?
- ❏ Yes
- ❏ No

How long do you want to live? _____

Why? _____

_____

Who is responsible for your health? _____

What will you be able to do as a non-smoker that you could not do
before? _____

_____

_____

What will you do with the money that you save? _____

_____

_____

Have you ever quit? If so, how did you do it and what happened?

_____

_____

Describe how you restarted: _____

_____

_____

_____

Why stop now? _____

_____

_____

_____

What are your concerns about quitting? _____

_____

_____

_____

What are your concerns about *not* quitting? _____

_____

_____

_____

Do you have any other addictions? _____

_____

Do you have any concerns about your weight? _____

_____

What is the strength of your desire to change? Please rate 1–100 _____

What are your expectations of hypnosis? _____

_____

_____

_____

# Appendix B

# *Example of Eating Questionnaire*

Name: _____

Sex: _____ Age: _____ Date of Birth: _____

Address: _____

_____

Home Phone: _____ Cell Phone: _____

**Weight History**

1.  Present weight: _____ Height: _____

2.  Describe your present weight: (circle one below)

    Very overweight     Slightly overweight     About average

3.  Are you dissatisfied with the way you look at this weight? (circle one below)

    Completely satisfied     Satisfied     Neutral     Dissatisfied     Very dissatisfied

4.  At what weight have you felt your best or do you think you would feel your best? _____

5.  How much weight would you like to lose? _____

6.  Do you feel your weight affects your daily activities?

    No effect     Some effect     Often interferes     Extreme effect

7.  Why do you want to lose weight at this time? _____

    _____

    _____

8. What are the attitudes of the following people about your attempt(s) to lose weight? (please check all that apply)

| | Negative (disapprove/resentful) | Indifferent (don't care) | Positive (encouraging/ understanding) |
|---|---|---|---|
| Husband | | | |
| Wife | | | |
| Children | | | |
| Parents | | | |
| Employer | | | |
| Friends | | | |

9. Do these attitudes affect your weight loss or gain? If yes, please describe: _____

_____

10. Indicate on the following table the periods in your life when you have been overweight. Where appropriate, list your maximum weight from each period and number of pounds you were overweight. Briefly describe any methods you used to lose weight in that five-year period (e.g., diet, shots, pills, etc.). Also, list any significant life events you feel were related to either your weight gain or loss (e.g., college tests, marriage, pregnancies, illnesses, etc.).

| Age | Max weight | Pounds overweight | Methods to lose weight | Significant events related to weight change |
|---|---|---|---|---|
| Birth | | | | |
| 0–5 | | | | |
| 5–10 | | | | |
| 10–15 | | | | |
| 15–20 | | | | |
| 20–25 | | | | |
| 25–30 | | | | |
| 30–35 | | | | |
| 35–40 | | | | |
| 40–45 | | | | |
| 45–50 | | | | |
| 50–55 | | | | |

11. How physically active are you?

Very Active    Active    Average    Inactive    Very inactive

12. What do you do for physical exercise and how often do you do it?

| Activity (e.g. swimming, jogging, dancing) | Frequency (daily, monthly, weekly) |
|---|---|
|  |  |
|  |  |
|  |  |
|  |  |
|  |  |
|  |  |
|  |  |
|  |  |

13. A number of different ways of losing weight are listed below. Please indicate which methods you have used by filling in the appropriate blanks:

| Method | Age(s) used | No. of times used | Max. weight lost | Comments (success/difficulties) |
|---|---|---|---|---|
| TOPS |  |  |  |  |
| Weight Watchers |  |  |  |  |
| Shots |  |  |  |  |
| Pills |  |  |  |  |
| Supervised diet |  |  |  |  |
| Unsupervised diet |  |  |  |  |
| Starvation |  |  |  |  |
| Behavior modification |  |  |  |  |
| Psychotherapy |  |  |  |  |
| Hypnosis |  |  |  |  |
| Other |  |  |  |  |

14. Which method did you use for the longest period of time?

_____

_____

15. Indicate any mood changes on the following checklist:

| | Not at all | A little bit | Moderately | Quite a bit | Extremely |
|---|---|---|---|---|---|
| Depressed, sad, feeling down, unhappy | | | | | |
| Anxious, nervous, restless, uptight | | | | | |
| Physically weak | | | | | |
| Elated, happy | | | | | |
| Easily irritated, annoyed, or angry | | | | | |
| Fatigued, worn out, tired all the time | | | | | |
| A lack of self-confidence | | | | | |

16. What usually goes wrong with your weight loss program?

_____

_____

**Medical History**

17. When did you last have a complete physical examination?

_____

18. Who is your current doctor? _____

19. What medical problems do you have at the present time?

_____

_____

20. What medication or drugs do you take regularly?

_____

_____

21. List any medications, drugs, or foods that you are allergic to:

_____

_____

22. List any hospitalizations or operations. Indicate how old you were at each hospital admission:

    **Age**        **Reason for hospitalization**

a. _____    _____

b. _____    _____

c. _____    _____

23. List any serious illnesses you have had which have not required hospitalization. Indicate how old you were during each illness:

    **Age**        **Illness**

a. _____    _____

b. _____    _____

c. _____    _____

24. Describe any of your medical problems that are complicated by excess weight:

_____

_____

_____

_____

25. How much alcohol do you usually drink per week?

_____

26. List any psychiatric contact, individual counseling, or marital counseling that you have had or are now having:

    **Age**        **Illness**

a. _____    _____

b. _____    _____

c. _____    _____

**Social History**

27. Circle the last year of school attended:

    1 2 3 4 5 6 7 8         9 10 11 12         1 2 3 4         M.A.         Ph.D.
    *Grade school*          *High school*      *College*

Other: _____

28. Describe your present occupation: _____

    _____

29. How long have you worked for your present employer?

    _____

30. Present marital status: (circle one)

    Single     Married     Divorced     Widowed     Separated     Engaged

31. Answer the following questions for each marriage:

Dates of marriages          _____   _____   _____

Date of termination(s)      _____   _____   _____

Reason (death, divorce, etc.) _____   _____   _____

Number of children          _____   _____   _____

32. Spouse's:

    Age _____ Weight _____ Height _____

33. Describe your spouse's occupation: _____

    _____

34. Describe your spouse's weight (circle one):

    Very          Slightly        About         Slightly        Very
    overweight    overweight      average       underweight     underweight

35. List your children's ages, sex, heights, and weights. Circle whether they are overweight, average, or underweight. Include any children from previous marriages, whether they are living with you or not:

| Age | Sex | Weight | Height | Overweight | | | | Underweight | |
|---|---|---|---|---|---|---|---|---|---|
| | | | | Very | Slightly | **Average** | Slightly | Very |
| | | | | Very | Slightly | **Average** | Slightly | Very |
| | | | | Very | Slightly | **Average** | Slightly | Very |
| | | | | Very | Slightly | **Average** | Slightly | Very |

36. Who lives at home with you? _____

37. Is your father living?     Yes     No

    Father's age now, or age at and cause of death:  _____

    _____

38. Is your mother living?     Yes     No

    Mother's age now, or age at and cause of death:  _____

    _____

39. Describe your father's occupation:  _____

    _____

40. Describe your mother's occupation:  _____

    _____

41. Describe your father's weight while you were growing up (circle one):

| Very overweight | Slightly overweight | About average | Slightly underweight | Very underweight |

42. Describe your mother's weight while you were growing up (circle one):

| Very overweight | Slightly overweight | About average | Slightly underweight | Very underweight |

43. List your siblings' ages, sex, present weights, and heights. Circle whether they are overweight, average, or underweight.

| Age | Sex | Weight | Height | Overweight | | | | Underweight | |
|---|---|---|---|---|---|---|---|---|---|
| | | | | Very | Slightly | **Average** | Slightly | Very |
| | | | | Very | Slightly | **Average** | Slightly | Very |
| | | | | Very | Slightly | **Average** | Slightly | Very |
| | | | | Very | Slightly | **Average** | Slightly | Very |

44. Please add any additional information you feel may be relevant to your weight problem. This includes interactions with your family and friends that might sabotage a weight loss program, and additional family or social history that you feel might help us understand your weight problem.

_____

_____

_____

_____

_____

_____

_____

_____

_____

# Resource List and Recommendations for Further Reading

## Alcohol and Problem Drinking

### Abstinence Approach

1. **Alcoholics Anonymous World Services (1976).** *Alcoholics anonymous "the Big book" (3rd Ed.).* **New York: Alcoholics Anonymous World Services.**
   This book is somewhat the "Bible" for AA 12-step programs. It describes the early origins of AA and the development of the steps that worked for the founders. Interestingly, other 12-step programs, such as Narcotics Anonymous (NA), Gamblers Anonymous (GA), Overeaters Anonymous (OA), and others, are all based on the original 12-steps of AA.

2. **Alcoholics Anonymous (1967).** *As Bill sees it: The A.A. way of life (selected writings of A.A.'s co-founder).* **New York: Alcoholics Anonymous World Services.**
   Interesting further reading for those who need to follow an abstinence program.

3. **Alcoholics Anonymous (1973).** *Came to believe.* **New York: Alcoholics Anonymous World Services.**
   Another book often recommended by A.A. "sponsors."

4. **Fanning, P. & O'Neil, J.T. (1996).** *The addiction workbook.* **Oakland, CA: New Harbinger.**
   This workbook gives some step-by-step guidance to working the steps.

5. **Joe McQ (1990).** *The steps we took.* **Little Rock, AR: August House.**
   Another book recommended by A.A. which reinforces the 12-step approach.

6. **Larsen, E. (1985). *Stage II recovery: Life beyond addiction.* San Francisco: Harper & Row.**
   This is an excellent reference book to help with relapse prevention. My story in Chapter 3 regarding the "Junkie driving my bus" came from this reference.

## Moderation Management Approach

1. **Alcohol Management: www.med.umich.edu/mfit/ alcoholmanagement/index.htm**
   This website offers support through in-person or telephone counseling by master's level counselors. I tend to recommend this one primarily for the client's further education about learning to drink moderately.

2. **Moderation Management: www.moderation.org**
   This website describes the theory and practice of moderate drinking and provides online support as well as information regarding developing meeting sites in a growing number of states.

   In California, such meetings take place in Orange County, San Diego, San Francisco, and Oakland. In New York, they are in Rochester, NYC-the Upper West Side & Midtown, and in W. Hampton Beach, Long Island. In D.C., they are in metro D.C. In Texas, there are meetings in Austin and Houston. There are also meetings in Colorado, Massachusetts, Minnesota, New Jersey, New Mexico, Virginia, Washington State, and Wisconsin, and one in Toronto. In addition, there are emerging meetings in Arizona, New Jersey, Oregon, Pennsylvania, and Virginia, and there are new ones being developed in New York City, Dallas, Wisconsin, and California.

3. **Rotgers, F., Kern, M., & Hoetzel, R. (2002). *Responsible drinking.* Oakland, CA: New Harbinger.**
   This book is supportive of the Moderation Management approach and how people can learn to drink responsibly.

4. **Vogler, R.E. & Bartz, W.R. (1982). *The better way to drink: Moderation and control of problem drinking.* Oakland, CA: New Harbinger.**
   Described by one reviewer as a responsible, conservatively written book on how problem drinkers whose bad habits are not too

far advanced can go about learning how to drink moderately. The authors also provide in an appendix a table for determining weight, number of drinks, and blood alcohol.

5.   **www.alcoholscreening.org**
     This website presents a drinking inventory for the individual to fill out, then provides him or her a percentage rate of people, by gender and overall, who drink less. For example, if the results are that the respondent drinks more frequently or in greater quantity than 90% of the people in the sample, this would surely suggest a significant problem. If 65% more, perhaps this finding would suggest a mild problem; 75 to 80%, moderate. (These are my interpretations; the site does not interpret the results.)

# Drug Abuse

1.   **The above-referenced books by Fanning and O'Neil (1996) and by Larsen (1985) are also recommended because they cover drug misuse/addiction as well as alcoholism.**

2.   **www.na.org**
     This is the website for Narcotics Anonymous World Services. Just as with A.A., the site can give information regarding meeting sites in various cities, or at least give telephone numbers to call. In most cities, there will be published a number in the telephone directory and a live voice or recording will give information about meeting sites. In smaller towns, where there are no N.A. chapters or very infrequent meetings, drug-addicted patients are referred to the local A.A. meetings, where participants are quite used to people not introducing themselves as an alcoholic, but rather as a drug addict, or both; for example, "Hello, my name is Frank. I am an alcoholic and drug addict." Anyone with an addiction who wants to follow the 12-step way is usually welcomed.

# Gambling

1.   **www.gamblersanonymous.org**
     This website will take one to the Gamblers Anonymous International Service located in Los Angeles, CA. At this website, there are phone numbers to talk to someone personally and an email

address: isomain@gamblersanonymous.org through which one can communicate.

Most cities that have casinos also have billboards advertising an "800" number for individuals to call if gambling has become a problem. There are also numbers listed in the telephone directory. In Baton Rouge, LA, for example, if the number is called, one gets a recording that says: "To speak with a volunteer, press 1; to hear a list of meeting places and times; press 2; to get information in the mail, press 3."

Once again, the above-referenced books for drug abuse (which were also listed for alcoholism) are helpful.

# Smoking Cessation

1.  **Hammond, D.C. (1990).** *Handbook of hypnotic suggestions and metaphors.* **New York: W.W. Norton.**
    There are a number of scripts in this edited work that have proved successful in working with smokers.

# Weight Loss

As was seen in Chapter 6, I am typically very permissive in what type of eating plan the client wants to employ, with the hypnosis helping them to stick to that plan. These include low-carbohydrate diets, low calorie diets, diabetic diets, Weight Watchers, the Zone Diet, and others. Some of the additional reading, depending on their choice of plans, follows:

1.  **Atkins, R.C. (2003).** *Atkins for life.* **New York: St. Martin's Press.**
    The earlier publications by Dr. Atkins were frowned upon by many nutritionists as being unhealthy over the long haul because of insufficient carbohydrates to fuel the body, especially during exercise. This version is more liberal in how carbohydrates are very limited at first, but healthy carbs are gradually worked back into the diet.

2.  **Sears, B. (1995).** *The zone.* **New York: HarperCollins.**
    **Sears, B. (1997).** *Mastering the zone.* **New York:**
    **HarperCollins.**
    These two books and the eating plan recommended seem to work especially well for individuals who commit to engage in vigorous exercise. Dr. Sears had worked with a number of athletes and noted how when an athlete is having a peak performance, he/she is said to be "in the zone." His approaches have to do with balancing amounts of fats, protein, and carbohydrates, based on one's activity level, to provide maximum hormonal balance.

3.  **Bays, J.C. (2009).** *Mindful eating: A guide to rediscovering a healthy and joyful relationship with food.* **New York: Random House.**
    I often tell clients that habit problems are "mindless." The Eastern monks who teach meditation have been talking about "mindfulness" for many centuries. It is only recently, however, that practitioners in the hypnotic field and in psychotherapy, in general, have begun stressing the importance of "mindfulness." This book focuses on the importance of mindfulness in our eating choices.

# Generic Scripts and Techniques

1.  **Allen, R.P. (2004).** *Scripts and strategies in hypnotherapy: The complete works.* **Bethel, CT: Crown House Publishing Ltd.**
    Although there are no specific scripts for alcohol, drugs, or gambling, this book is listed in the reference section because I occasionally reference using his "generic control habit" script with some clients.

2.  **Hammond, D.C. (1990).** *Handbook of hypnotic suggestions and metaphors.* **New York: W.W. Norton.**
    This excellent compilation of techniques and scripts provides no specific scripts for alcohol, gambling, or drug treatments, but has hypnotic techniques and generic scripts that can be applied. Most newcomers to ASCH find this an invaluable addition to their beginning to do clinical hypnosis.

3. **Havens, R. & Walters, C. (1989).** *Hypnotherapy scripts: A neo-Erickson approach to persuasive healing.* **New York: Bruner/Mazel.**
   This book also presents interesting techniques and scripts, albeit none specifically addressing alcohol, drugs, or gambling.

4. **Psychology of Addictive Behaviors.**
   This is the journal of Division 50 of the American Psychological Association (Addictions).

   More information may also be found at APA Division 50's website: www.apa.org/divisions/div50/.

# References

Allen, R.P. (2004). *Scripts and strategies in hypnotherapy: The complete works.* Bethel, CT: Crown House Publishing Ltd.

Bandler, R. & Grinder, J. (1976). *Frogs into Princes: Neuro Linguistic Programming.* Moab, UT: Real People Press.

Cautela, J.R.(1966). Treatment of compulsive behavior by covert sensitization. *Psychological Record, 16,* 33–41.

Chapman, R.A. (2008). The use of hypnosis in cognitive behavioral therapy. *American Society of Clinical Hypnosis Newsletter, Summer 2008.*

Cheek, D.B. & LeCron, L.M. (1968). *Clinical hypnotherapy.* New York: Grune & Stratton.

Citrenbaum, C.M., King, M.E., & Cohen, W.I. (1985). *Modern clinical hypnosis for habit control.* New York: W.W. Norton.

Crasilneck, H.B. & Hall, J.A. (1990). Suggestions for smoking cessation. In D.C. Hammond, *Handbook of hypnotic suggestions and metaphors* (pp. 416–417). New York: W.W. Norton.

DePiano, F. (2004). Division 30 Bulletin. *Psychological Hypnosis, 13(3),* 16–17.

de Shazer, S. (1988). *Clues: Investigating solutions in brief therapy.* New York: W.W. Norton.

Erickson, M.H. (1976).The interpersonal technique for symptom correction and pain control. *American Journal of Clinical Hypnosis, 8,* 198–200.

Ewin, D.M. & Eimer, B.N. (2006). *Ideomotor signals for rapid hypnoanalysis: A how-to manual.* Springfield, IL: Charles Thomas.

Ewin, D.M. (2008) Ideomotor signaling in the treatment of psychosomatic illness. Workshop sponsored by the New Orleans Society for Clinical Hypnosis, New Orleans, LA.

Feamster, J.H. & Brown, J.E. (1963). Hypnotic aversion to alcohol: three-year follow-up of one patient. *American Journal of Clinical Hypnosis, 6,* 164–166.

Festinger, L. (1957). *A theory of cognitive dissonance.* Stanford, CA: Stanford University Press.

Flemons, D. (2002). *Of one mind.* New York: W.W. Norton (p. 173).

Garver, R.E. (1990). In D.C. Hammond, *Handbook of hypnotic suggestions and metaphors* (p. 61). New York: W.W. Norton.

Glasser, W. (1984). *Take effective control of your life.* New York: Harper & Row, Publishers, Inc.

Gregg, D.M. (1973). Analeptic circle. In ASCH, Education and Research Foundation, *A syllabus on hypnosis and a handbook of therapeutic suggestions* (pp. 25–26).

Grinder, J. & Bandler, R. (1976). *The Structure Of Magic II: A Book About Communication and Change.* Palo Alto, CA: Science and Behavior Books.

Haley, J. (1985). *Conversations with Milton H. Erickson: Vol I: Changing individuals.* New York: Triangle Press.

Hammond, D.C. (1990). *Handbook of hypnotic suggestions and metaphors.* New York: W.W. Norton.

Hartland, J. (1966). *Medical and dental hypnosis.* London: Tindale and Cassell (pp 191–192).

Havens, R. & Walters, C. (1989). *Hypnotherapy scripts: A neo-Erickson approach to persuasive healing.* New York: Bruner/Mazel.

Kroger, W.S. and Fezler, W.D. (1976). *Hypnosis and behavior modification: Imagery conditioning.* Philadelphia, Toronto: J.B. Lippincott Company.

Larsen, E. (1984). *Stage II recovery: Life beyond addiction.* San Francisco: Harper.

LaScola, R. (1973). Treating the teen-age drug abuser with hypnosis. *A syllabus on hypnosis and a handbook of therapeutic suggestions.* ASCH Educational and Research Foundation.

Lemonick, M.D. & Park, A. (2007). The science of addiction. *Time, July* 16, 42–48.

Meichenbaum, D. (1977). *Cognitive-behavior modification: An integrative approach.* New York: Plenum Press.

Mutter, C.B. & Crasilneck, H. (2007). Hypnosis and pain control. Workshop presented at ASCH/SCEH, Dallas, TX.

Myss, C. (2002). *Sacred contracts: Awakening your divine potential.* New York: Three Rivers Press.

Pieper, M.H. & Pieper, W.J. (2003). *Addicted to unhappiness.* New York: McGraw-Hill.

Poulos, L. & Smith, M. (1998). Sports medicine. Workshop presented at 40th annual ASCH Workshops, Ft. Worth, TX.

Rossi, E.L. (1980). *The collected papers of Milton Erickson on Hypnosis, Vol I–IV.* New York: Irvington.

Rossi, E.L. & Cheek, D.B. (1988). *Mind-body therapy: Methods of ideodynamic healing in hypnosis.* New York: W.W. Norton.

Rotgers, F., Kern, M. & Hoeltzel, R. (2002). *Responsible drinking.* Oakland, CA: New Harbinger.

Shapiro, M. (2005). Customizing hypnosis for your practice. Workshop presented at 47th Annual ASCH Workshops, St. Louis, MO.

Sobell, M.B. & Sobell, L.C. (1993). *Problem drinkers: Guided self-change treatment.* New York: Guilford.

Spiegel, H. & Spiegel, D. (1978). *Trance and treatment: Clinical uses of hypnosis.* New York: Basic Books.

Stock, M. (1990). Aversive metaphor for smoking. In Hammonds (Ed), *Handbook of hypnotic suggestions and metaphors.* New York: W.W. Norton (pp. 423–425).

Torem, M. (2007). Strategies for weight control incorporating hypnosis. Workshop presented at ASCH/SCEH Workshops, Dallas, TX.

Tramontana, J. (2005). Hypnotherapy and hypnosis as an adjunctive technique in psychotherapy. CEU Seminar presented at Gulfport, MS VA.

Whitfield, C. (1987). *Healing the child within: Discovery and recovery for adult children of dysfunctional families.* Deerfield Beach, FL: Health Communications, Inc.

Williams, R.L. & Tramontana, J. (1975). A rural survey: The middle aged pill popper. *Rushes, 2(4),* Mississippi Clearinghouse for Drug Misuse Information.

Williams, R.L. & Tramontana, J. (1977). The evaluation of occupational alcoholism programs. In C. J. Schramm (Ed.), *Alcoholism and its treatment in industry*. Baltimore, MD: Johns Hopkins University Press.

Wright, M.E. (1987). *Clinical practice of hypnotherapy*. New York: Guilford.

Yarnell, R. (1996). *Ultimate hypnosis practice system*. Austin: Yarnell Publishing.

Yarnell, R. (1998). Hypnosis marketing seminar, Orlando, FL.

Zarren, J.I. & Eimer, B.N. (2002). *Brief cognitive hypnosis: facilitating the change of dysfunctional behavior*. New York: Springer.

Zeig, J. (2005). A "states" model: A phenomenological perspective to hypnotherapy. Presentation at 47th Annual ASCH Workshops, St. Louis, MO.

Zimberoff, D. (1999). Heart-centered therapies. Workshop, The Wellness Institute, New Orleans.

# Index

abstinence model
    in addiction recovery, 22–23,
        110–111
    for addictive personalities, 39–40
    for drug addiction/abuse, 44
    resources, 129–130
    smoking cessation, 77, 85
    v. controlled drinking, 34–36
acting-out cycle, 5, 56
*Addicted to Unhappiness* (Pieper), 46
"addictive personality," 39–40
addictive-compulsive behavior, 27
addicts. *see also* drug abuse/
        addiction; food addiction/
        compulsions; gambling
        addiction
    "addictive personality," 39–40
    attraction of hypnosis, 21
    cross-addiction, 48, 65, 113
    treatment choices, 21
"affect-bridge," 2, 97, 98–99
alcohol abuse/dependency. *see also*
        controlled drinking
    abstinence model, 22–23
    Alcohol Management, 33–34, 130
    alcohol screening, 22
    Alcoholics Anonymous, ix, 19, 20,
        22, 27, 44, 129
    hypnosis treatment, 19–23
    MM model, 20–22
    negative transference, ix
    rehabilitation approaches, 20
    treatment choices, 20–22
    treatment plans, individualized,
        20–21
Alcohol Management, 33–34, 130
alcohol screening, 22
Alcoholics Anonymous (AA), ix, 19,
        20, 22, 27, 44, 129
Allen, Roger P., 60

amends, 30–33
American Society for Clinical
        Hypnosis (ASCH), v, 8, 116
anxiety/stress reduction, 1, 12, 43, 47
aversive stimuli technique, 2, 78–82,
        110–111

bankroll, 56
beach/ocean scene imagery, 8, 10, 25
behavior modification, 74–77
betting questionnaire, 53–54
blackouts, 42
body image, 93, 94
breathing exercises
    deep, 15–16, 23–24, 29, 71, 92
    diaphragmatic breathing, 10,
        15–16
busters symbol, 94

Chantrix, 85
Cheek, David, 3, 62
coaching metaphor, 3–4
cocaine, 44–45, 48–49, 55, 113
codependent behavior, 27–28, 98
cognitive-behavioral techniques/
        approaches, x, 33, 60–62
collapsing anchors, 66–67, 82–83, 110
*Collected Papers of Milton H. Erickson
        on Hypnosis, The* (Rossi), x
comps, 57, 58
compulsive behavior, ix, 27, 53, 66,
        113
conflict, 63
control switch visualization, 46–47
controlled drinking
    Alcohol Management, 33–34, 130
    hypnotic suggestions, 34–35
    MM approach, 21–22, 33, 130–131
    strategies, 20, 34
    v. abstinence, 34–36

devious behavior, 55
Gamblers Anonymous (GA), 27,
58–59
"gambler's fallacy," 58
gambling "lingo," 56–58
"good players," 60–61
help lines for problem gamblers,
58
hypnotic induction, 63
managed approach, failure of, 65
metaphors/stories, 60–61
muscle testing technique, 62–63
on-line poker, 53
past experience triggers, 64
psychological issues, 65–66
questionnaire, 53–54
resources, 131–132
therapeutic techniques, 60
gambling "lingo," 56–58
generalization effect, 12–13, 25, 71
"Generic Habit Control" (Allen), 60
generic scripts and techniques,
133–134
glove anesthesia, 13
goal-directed treatment, 21
God, 28–32
"good players" (gambling), 60–61

habits, 73–74
"healing the wounded child within,"
x, 98
healthy relationships, 41–42
high rollers, 56–57, 61
higher power, 28–31
house (gambling facility), 57, 58
hypnoprojection, 2, 35, 97
hypnosis/hypnotherapy overview,
1–2, 6–9, 23
hypnotic enhancement, x
hypnotic regression. *see also*
uncovering
for "self-sabotage," 32, 35, 46, 60
for smoking cessation, 71–72, 78
for weight problems, 105

hypnotic states, x–xi, 12–13
hypnotic suggestibility, tests of, 7–9,
91
hypnotic suggestions, 24, 34–35, 78,
92–95
"hypnotically enhanced," x
hypnotizability, 8, 14

ideomotor techniques, 3, 61–65,
109–110
imagery, 9–10, 15, 23–24, 35–36
impulse-control disorders, 113
individualized treatment plans,
20–21, 44
induction techniques. *see* elicitation/
induction of hypnotic state
*Insider, The* (film), 73
Internet addiction, 113

key words, 12, 25–26, 102

Larsen, Earnie, 45
lines of credit, 56–57
log jam metaphor, 25–27, 102–104

maladaptive behavior, 40, 46, 55, 110,
112
marijuana, 2, 43, 48–49
markers, 57
marketing/packaging techniques
payment plans, 112
smoking cessation, 69–70, 84–85
weight loss, 87–88
master control room technique,
46–47
meditation, 30
meditational statements, 76
meditational statements, 76, 81–82,
83
food addiction/compulsions, 95
metaphors/stories
coaching metaphor, 3–4
"good players" (gambling), 60–61
log jam metaphor, 25–27, 102–104